Pathophysiologic Word Book

Diane L. Shaw

**Springhouse
Word Book Series**

Springhouse Corporation
Springhouse, Pennsylvania

© Copyright 1992 by
Springhouse Corporation
1111 Bethlehem Pike
Springhouse, Pennsylvania 19477

All rights reserved. No part of this book may be reproduced, stored in a retrieval system or transmitted in any form or by any means, electronic, mechanical, photocopying, recording or otherwise, without written permission from the publisher, except for brief quotations embodied in critical articles and reviews.

Printed in the United States of America

Library of Congress Catalog Card Number: 89-051118

ISBN: 0-87434-424-7

SWB 8-010891

**This book is affectionately dedicated to
my support system:
Allen, Julie, and Paula**

Preface

This word book is a collection of words, phrases, and abbreviations related to the dysfunction of physiologic processes that occur as a result of infection, heredity, and/or the environment. Also included is the binomial nomenclature of a large variety of microbial pathogens. As a further aid, the text is extensively cross referenced. For example, a condition such as Volkmann's contracture may be located from either word:

    Volkmann's contracture
    contracture
        Volkmann's.

A complete list of diseases may be found at the back of the book.

A

AAA (abdominal aortic aneurysm)
AAR (aortic arch syndrome)
AB (asthmatic bronchitis)
Abadie's sign
abalienation
abarognosis
abasia
- a. astasia
- a. atactica
- choreic a.
- paralytic a.
- paroxysmal trepidant a.
- spastic a.
- a. trepidans

abdominal
- a. angina
- a. aortic aneurysm (AAA)
- a. apoplexy
- a. epilepsy
- a. migraine
- a. muscle deficiency syndrome (prune-belly syndrome)
- a. seizure equivalent (abdominal epilepsy)
- a. testis

abducent paralysis
aberrant
- a. ductule
- a. pancreas
- a. renal vessels
- a. tissue

aberration
- chromatic a.

aberration *(continued)*
- chromosome a.
- dioptric a.
- distantial a.
- heterosomal a.
- homosomal a.
- meridional a.
- newtonian a.
- penta-X chromosomal a.
- spherical a.
- tetra-X chromosomal a.
- triple-X chromosomal a.

abetalipoproteinemia (Bassen-Kornzweig syndrome)
abiotrophy
ABL (abetalipoproteinemia)
ablatio
- a. placentae
- a. retinae

ablepharia
ablepsia
abomasitis
abortion
- afebrile a.
- ampullar a.
- artifical a.
- cervical a.
- complete a.
- contagious a.
- criminal a.
- habitual a.
- imminent a.
- incomplete a.
- induced a.
- inevitable a.

Additional Entries
_____
_____
_____
_____
_____

abortion *(continued)*
    infected a.
    missed a.
    septic a.
    spontaneous a.
    threatened a.
    tubal a.
abortive infection
abortive poliomyelitis
Abrikosov's or Abrikosoff's tumor (granular-cell myoblastoma)
abruptio placentae
abscess
    acute a.
    alveolar a.
    amebic a.
    apical a.
    Bartholin's a.
    Brodie's a.
    cerebral a.
    chronic a.
    epidural a.
    Kogoj's a.
    Monro's a.
    perinephric a.
    subdiaphragmatic a.
    subhepatic a.
    tubo-ovarian a.
absence attack or seizure (petit mal seizure)
Absidia
    A. corymbifera
    A. ramosa
absolute
    a. glaucoma
    a. hyperopia
    a. scotoma

absorption atelectasis (obstructive atelectasis)
abstinence delirium
abulia
abulomania
acalcicosis
acalculia
acampsia
acanthamebiasis
Acanthamoeba
    A. castellani
    A. hartmannella
acanthesthesia
Acanthocephala
acanthocephaliasis
Acanthocheilonema
    A. perstans
    A. streptocerca
acanthocyte
acanthocytosis
acanthokeratoma (keratoacanthoma)
acantholysis
acanthoma
    a. adenoides cysticum
    basal cell a.
    a. verrucosa seborrheica
acanthorrhexis
acanthosis
    a. nigricans
acapnia (hypocapnia)
acardia
acardiac
acardiotrophia
acariasis
acarid
Acarina
acarinosis

Additional Entries

acarodermatitis
    a. urticarioides (grain itch)
acarophobia
Acarus
    A. folliculorum
    A. gallinae
    A. hordei
    A. rhyzoplypticus hyacinthi
    A. scabiei
    A. siro
acatalasemia, acatalasaemia
acatalasia
acatamathesia
acataphasia
acathexia
acathexis
ACC (adenoid cystic carcioma)
accidental albuminuria (false proteinuria)
accident neurosis (traumatic neurosis)
accommodation paralysis
accoucheur's hand
acelomate
acenesthesia, acoenaesthesia
acephalocyst
acephalous
    a. dibrachius
    a. dipus
    a. monobrachius
    a. monopus
    a. paracephalus
    a. sympus
Acetobacter
    A. aceti
    A. melanogenus
    A. oxydans

Acetobacter *(continued)*
    A. rancens
    A. roseus
    A. suboxydans
    A. xylinum
acetonemia (ketonemia)
acetonuria (ketonuria)
achalasia
    biliary a.
    esophageal a.
    pelvirectal a.
    sphincteral a.
Achard-Thiers syndrome
ache
acheirus, achirus
achillobursitis
achillodynia
achlorhydria
achloropsia
Acholeplasma laidlawii
acholia
acholuria
acholuric jaundice
achondrogenesis
achondroplasia
achondroplastic dwarf
Achorion
    A. schoenleini
    A. violaceum
achromacyte
achromasia
achromat
achromatopsia
achromatosis (achromasia)
achromatous
achromaturia
achromia
achromia cutis

Additional Entries

achromic
Achromobacter
Achromobacteraceae
achromotrichia
achylanemia, achylanaemia
achylia
    a. gastrica
achylous
achymia
Acidaminococcus
    A. fermentans
acidaminuria (aminoaciduria)
acidemia
    argininosuccinic a.
    glutaric a.
    isovaleric a.
    methylmalonic a.
    propionic a.
acid intoxication
acidosis
    compensated a.
    diabetic a.
    hypercapnic a.
    hyperchloremic a.
    metabolic a.
    metabolic a., compensated
    nonrespiratory a.
    renal hyperchloremia a.
    renal tubular a.
    respiratory a.
    respiratory a., compensated
    starvation a.
    uremic a.
acidotic
acid tide
aciduria
    acetoacetic a.

aciduria *(continued)*
    argininosuccinic a.
    beta-aminoisobutyric a.
    ethylmalonic-adipic a.
    glutaric a.
    methylmalonic a.
    orotic a.
    pyroglutamic a.
acinesia (akinesia)
Acinetobacter
    A. anitratus
    A. calcoaceticus
    A. lwoffi
    A. parapertussis
acinic
    a. cell adenocarcinoma
    a. cell tumor
acladiosis
Acladium
aclasia
aclasis
    diaphyseal a.
    tarsoepiphyseal a.
aclastic
acleistocardia
acne
    a. atrophica
    bromide a.
    a. cachecticorum
    chlorine a.
    a. coagminata
    common a. (vulgaris)
    a. conglobata
    a. cosmetica
    a. cystica (folliculitis decalvans)
    a. detergicans

Additional Entries

acne *(continued)*
    epidemic a. (keratosis follicularis contagiosa)
    a. estivalis
    excoriated a. (a. excoriee des filles, a. excoriee des jeunes filles)
    a. frontalis
    a. fulminans
    halogen a.
    a. indurata
    infantile a.
    iodide a.
    a. keloid
    Mallorca a.
    a. mechanica
    a. medicamentosa
    a. neonatorum
acneform
acneform drug eruptions
acnegen
acneiform (acneform)
aconuresis
acoprosis
acorea
acoria, akoria
acostate
acousma
acousmatagnosis
acoustic
    a. neurilemmoma (schwannoma)
    a. neuroma
acousticomotor epilepsy
acousticophobia
acquired
    a. agammaglobulinemia
    a. hemolytic anemia

acquired *(continued)*
    a. immune deficiency syndrome (AIDS)
    a. resistance
acrania
acraturesis
Acremonium
acroanesthesia
acroarthritis
acroasphyxia
acroataxia
acrobrachycephaly
acrocephalopolysyndactyly
acrocephaly
acrochordon
acrocyanosis (Crocq's disease)
acrodermatitis
    a. chronica atrophicans
    a. continua
    a. hiemalis
    a. perstans
acrodolichomelia
acrodynia
acroedema
acroesthesia
acrohyperhidrosis
acrohypothermy
acrokeratosis
    a. verruciformis
acrokinesis
acromegalic arthritis
acromegaloid
acromegaly (Marie's syndrome)
acrometagenesis
acromyotonia
acroneuropathy
acroneurosis
acronyx

Additional Entries

acroosteolysis
acropachy
acropachyderma
acroparalysis
acroparesthesia
acropathology
acropathy
acroposthitis
acroscleroderma
acrosclerosis
acrospiroma
Acrotheca pedrosoi
Acrothesium floccosum
acrotrophoneurosis
actinic
    a. carcinoma
    a. dermatosis
    a. keratoconjunctivitis
    a. keratosis
Actinobacillus
    A. actinomycetemcomitans
    A. lignieresii
    A. mallei
    A. pseudomallei
actinodermatitis
Actinomadura
    A. madurae
    A. pelletierii
Actinomyces
    A. bovis
    A. congolensis
    A. eriksonii
    A. israelii
    A. muris
    A. muris-ratti
    A. naeslundii
    A. necrophorus
    A. odontolyticus

Actinomyces *(continued)*
    A. rhusiopathiae
    A. vinaceus
    A. viscosus
Actinomycetaceae
Actinomycetales
actinomycete
actinomycetoma
actinomycoma
actinomycosis
actinomycotic
    a. mycetoma
actinoneuritis
Actinoplanes
Actinopoda
acute
    a. abdomen
    a. abscess
    a. appendicitis
    a. ascending myelitis
    a. bacterial endocarditis
    a. bacterial pharyngitis
    a. brain syndrome
    a. bronchitis
    a. cardiovascular disease
    a. cerebellar ataxia
    a. disseminated encephalomyelitis
    a. duodenal ileus (arteriomesenteric ileus, gastromesenteric ileus)
    a glomerulonephritis
    a. inflammation
    a. intermittent porphyria
    a. interstitial nephritides
    a. leukemia
    a. mastitis

Additional Entries

acute *(continued)*
    a. monocytic
      (monoblastic) leukemia
    a. myelitis
    a. myelocytic leukemia
    a. myelomonocytic
      leukemia
    a. necrotizing
      hemorrhagic
      encephalomyelitis
      (acute hemorrhagic
      leukoencephalitis of
      Weston Hurs
    a. necrotizing ulcerative
      gingivitis
    a. organic brain syndrome
      (acute brain syndrome)
    a. peritonitis
    a. pharyngitis
    a. promyelocytic leukemia
    a. pyelonephritis
    a. rejection
    a. renal failure
    a. respiratory disease
      (ARD)
    a. rhinitis of the newborn
    a. splenitis
    a. toxic encephalopathy
    a. traumatic subdural
      hygroma
    a. tubular necrosis (ATN)
    a. undifferentiated
      leukemia
    a. yellow atrophy
acyanoblepsia (acyanopsia)
acyanopsia
acyanotic
acyclia
acyesia
acystia
adacrya
adactylia
adactylous
adactyly
adamantinocarcinoma
adamantinoma
    pituitary a.
adamantinomatoid
    craniopharyngioma
Adams-Stokes syndrome
    (Stokes-Adams syndrome)
adaptation disease
addisonian
    a. crisis (adrenal crisis)
addisonism
Addison's
    anemia (pernicious
      anemia)
    disease or syndrome
      (asthenia pigmentosa,
      melanoma suprarenale)
adenalgia
adenasthenia
adenitis
    acute epidemic infectious
      a.
    acute salivary a.
    cervical a.
    mesenteric a.
    phlegmonous a.
    a. tropicalis
adenoacanthoma
adenoameloblastoma
adenoangiosarcoma
adenocarcinoma
    acinic cell a.

Additional Entries

adenocarcinoma *(continued)*
    alveolar a.
    anaplastic a.
    bronchiolar a.
    clear cell a.
    colloid a.
    follicular a.
    gelatinous a.
    Hurthle cell a.
    infiltrating duct a.
    inflammatory a.
    a. in-situ
    lobular a.
    medullary a.
    mesonephric a.
    mucinous a.
    papillary a.
    sebaceous a.
    signet ring a.
    sweat gland a.
    trabecular a.
    undifferentiated a.
adenocarcinomatosis
adenocellulitis
adenochondroma
adenocystic
    a. carcinoma
    a. disease
adenocystoma
    a. lymphomatosum
        (Warthin's tumor)
adenofibroma
adenofibrosis
adenoid cystic carcinoma
adenoiditis
adenoleiomyoma
   (adenomyoma)
adenolipoma
adenolymphoma
adenoma
    acidophilic a.
    adnexal a.
    adrenocortical a.
    apocrine a.
    basophilic a.
    bile duct a.
    bronchial a.
    ceruminous a.
    chief cell a.
    chromophobe a.
    clear cell a.
    colloid a.
    embryonal a.
    a. destruens
    eosinophil a.
    fetal a.
    follicular a.
    Hurthle cell a.
    islet cell a.
    liver cell a.
    macrofollicular a.
    a. malignum (malignant
       a.)
    microfollicular a.
    oncocytic a.
    oxyphil a.
    papillary a.
    Pick's tubular a.
    polypoid a.
    a. sebaceum (Pringle's
       adenoma sebaceum)
    sweat gland a.
    trabecular a.
    tubular a.
    villous a.
adenomalacia

Additional Entries

adenomatoid
   a. tumor
adenomatosis
adenomatous
   a. goiter (nodular goiter, multiple colloid adenomatous goiter)
   a. hyperplasia
   a. polyp
adenomyoma (adenoleiomyoma)
adenomyosalpingitis (isthmic nodular salpingitis)
adenomyosarcoma
adenomyosis
adenomyxochondrosarcoma
adenomyxoma
adenomyxosarcoma
adenopathy
adenopharyngitis
adenosarcoma
adenosis
   blunt duct a.
   breast a.
   fibrosing a.
   sclerosing a.
   vaginal a.
adenosquamous carcinoma
adenovirus (APC virus)
adhesion
   amniotic a.
   fibrinous a.
   fibrous a.
   sublabial a.
adhesive
   a. arachnoiditis
   a. chronic pachymeningitis

adhesive *(continued)*
   a. pericardiomediastinitis
   a. pericarditis
adiadochokinesis
adiaspiromycosis
Adie's pupil (pseudo Argyll Robertson pupil)
Adie's syndrome
adipokinesis
adipoma (lipoma)
adiponecrosis
   a. neonatorum
adipose gynism (Simpson's syndrome in females)
adiposis
   a. cerebralis
   a. dolorosa (Dercum's disease)
   a. hepatica
   a. tuberosa simplex
   a. universalis
adipositis
adiposity
adiposogenital dystrophy
adiposuria
adipsia
adipsy (adipsia)
adnauseam
adnexal
   a. adenoma
   a. carcinoma
adnexitis (salpingo-oophoritis)
adolescent goiter
adrenal
   a. apoplexy
   a. cortical insufficiency
   a. crisis (addisonian crisis)

Additional Entries

adrenal *(continued)*
    a. virilism syndrome
       (adrenogenital
       syndrome)
adrenalitis
adrenocortical obesity
adrenocorticoid adenoma of the
    ovary
adrenogential syndrome
adrenosympathetic syndrome
    (Page's syndrome)
adrenotropism
adromia
ADS (antibody deficiency
    syndrome)
adtorsion
adult Fanconi syndrome
adventitious albuminuria
adynamia
    a. episodica hereditaria
       (Gamstorp's disease)
adynamic ileus
Aedes
    A. aegypti
    A. albopictus
    A. cinereus
    A. flavescens
    A. leucocelaenus
    A. scutellaris
       pseudoscutellaris
    A. sollicitans
    A. spencerii
    A. taeniorhynchus
aelurophilia (galeophilia)
aelurophobia (galeophobia)
aeluropsis
aeremia, aeraemia
aeroatelectasis

Aerobacter (Enterobacter)
    A. aerogenes (Enterobacter
       aerogenes)
    A. cloacae
    A. lipolyticus
    A. liquefaciens
    A. subgroup A, B, C
aerobe
aerobic
aerocele
Aerococcus
    A. viridans
Aeromonas
    A. hydrophila
    A. liquefaciens
    A. punctata
    A. salmonicida
    A. shigelloides
aeroneurosis
aerootitis (barotitis)
aeropathy
aerophagia
aerophobia
aerosinusitis (barosinusitis)
aerosis
aerotropism
AFB (acid-fast bacilli)
affective disorder
afferent loop syndrome
AFIB (atrial fibrillation)
afibrinogenemia
AFL (atrial flutter)
aflatoxin
African
    A. lymphoma (Burkitt's
       lymphoma)
    A. sleeping sickness
    A. tick borne fever

Additional Entries

African *(continued)*
    A. trypanosomiasia
agalactia
agammaglobulinemia
Agamodistomum
    ophthalmobium
Agamonema
Agamonematodum migrans
aganglionic megacolon
    (Hirschsprung's disease)
aganglionosis
Agarbacterium
agenesis
agenitalism
agenosomia
ageusia
ageustic aphasia
aggressive behavior disorder
agitated dementia
agitographia
agitophasia
AGL (acute granulocytic
    leukemia)
aglandular
aglobulia
aglobuliosis
aglobulism
aglomerular
aglossia
aglutition (dysphagia)
aglycemia
agnathus
agnogenic
    A. myeloid metaplasia
agnosia
agomphiasis
agomphious
agonadism

agonal intussusception
agoraphobia
agranulocytic angina
agranulocytosis
agranuloplasia
agraphia
Agrobacterium
agrypnotic
aguc
    a. cake spleen
agyria
AH (arterial hypertension)
AHA (aquired hemolytic anemia)
AI (aortic insufficiency)
aichmophobia
AID (acute infectious disease)
AIDS (acquired immune
    deficiency syndrome)
AIHA (autoimmune hemolytic
    anemia)
ailurophilia (galeophilia)
ailurophobia (galeophobia)
air
    a. embolism
    a. hunger (Kussmaul's
        respiration)
    a. sickness
air-borne infection
Ajellomyces
    A. dermatitidis
akathisia
akinesia
akinesthesia
akinetic
    a. epilepsy
    a. mutism
    a. seizure
alalia

Additional Entries

alaninemia
alaninuria
alatus
Albers-Schonberg's disease
  (osteopetrosis)
albiduria
albinism
albino
albinotic
Albright's syndrome
albuginitis
albuminocytologic dissociation
albuminuria
albumosuria
Alcaligenes
    A. bookeri
    A. bronchosepticus
    A. denitrificans
    A. faecalis
    A. marshallii
    A. metalcaligenes
    A. odorans
    A. recti
    A. viscolactis
alcaptonuria
alcoholic
  a. delirium
  a. myopathy
alcoholism (acute alcoholism)
Alder-Reilly anomaly
Alder's anomaly
aldosteronism
  (hyperaldosteronism)
Aldrich syndrome (Wiskott-
  Aldrich syndrome)
aleukemic
  a. granulocytic leukemia
  a. leukemia

aleukemic *(continued)*
  a. lymphocytic leukemia
  a. monocytic leukemia
  a. myelosis
aleukocytosis
Alexander's disease
alexia
algid stage
Alginobacter
Alginomonas
algospasm
alimentary
  a. glucosuria
  a. lipemia
alkalemia
alkalosis
  compensated a.
  hypokalemic a.
  metabolic a.
  nonrespiratory a.
  potassium a.
  respiratory a.
allantoic cyst
allergic
  a. conjunctivitis
  a. contact dermatitis
  a. encephalitis
  a. encephalomyelitis
  a. granulomatosis
  a. granulomatous angiitis
  a. neuritis
  a. purpura
  a. reaction
  a. rhinitis
  a. urticaria
allergy
Allescheria
    A. boydii

Additional Entries

allescheriosis
alloalbuminemia
allochezia
Allodermanyssus
    A. sanguineus
alopecia
    a. areata
    a. cicatrisata
    a. congenitalis
    a. mucinosa
    a. prematura
    a. syphilitica
    a. universalis
alphatoxin
alphavirus
altitude
    a. alkalosis
    a. anoxia
    a. sickness
aluminosis
alusia (hallucination)
alveolar
    a. abscess
    a. adenocarcinoma
    a. capillary block
        syndrome
    a. carcinoma (bronchiolar
        carcinoma)
    a. cyst
    a. proteinosis
    a. rhabdomyosarcoma
    a. soft part sarcoma
alveolitis
alveoloclasia
alymphocytosis
alysmus
Alzheimer's
    A's disease

Alzheimer's *(continued)*
    A's plaque (argyrophil
        plaque)
Amanita
    A. muscaria
    A. pantherina
    A. phalloides
    A. rubescens
    A. verna
    A. virosa
amasesis
amastia
amathophobia
amaurosis
    a. fugax
    a. partialis fugax
amaurotic
    a. familial idiocy
Amblyoma
amblyopia
    a. ex anopsia
ameba, amoeba
    coprozoic a.
amebiasis, amoebiasis
    a. cutis
amebic, amoebic
    a. abscess
    a. colitis
    a. dysentery
    a. gangrene
    a. granuloma (ameboma)
    a. hepatitis
    a. meningoencephalitis
ameboma
amelanotic melanoma
amelia
ameloblastic
    a. fibroma

Additional Entries

ameloblastic *(continued)*
    a. hemangioma
    a. neurilemoma
    a. odontoma
    a. sarcoma
ameloblastoma
    calcifying a.
amelogenesis imperfecta
amenorrhea
amentia
American mucocutaneous
    leishmaniasis
American spotted fever (Rocky
    Mountain spotted fever)
ametria
amianthinopsy
aminoacidemia
aminoaciduria
ammonemia
ammoniuria
amnesia
    hysterical a.
    transient a.
amnionitis
amniorrhea
amniotic
    a. adhesions
    a. cyst
amniotitis
Amoeba
    A. buccalis
    A. cachexica
    A. coli
    A. coli mitis
    A. dentalis
    A. dysenteriae
    A. histolytica
    A. limax

Amoeba *(continued)*
    A. meleagridis
    A. urinae granulata
    A. urogenitalis
    A. verrucosa
amphiarthrosis
amphicrania
Amphimerus
amphixenoses
amphodiplopia
ampullar pregnancy
ampullary aneurysm
amychophobia
amyelia
amyelonic
amylasuria
amylodyspepsia
amyloid
    a. degeneration
    a. tumor
amyloidosis
    diffuse a.
    familial primary systemic
      a.
    focal a.
    primary a.
    secondary a.
amylopectinosis (Andersen's
    disease)
amylorrhea
amyoplasia
    a. congenita
amyostasia
amyotaxia
amyotonia
    a. congenita
amyotrophia spinalis
    progressiva

Additional Entries

amyotrophic lateral sclerosis
amyotrophy
    diabetic a.
    neuralgic a.
amyxia
An (anisometropia)
anacmesis
anacousia, anacusia
anacrotic pulse
anacrotic shoulder
anaerobe
    falcultative a.
    obligate a.
anaerobic
    a. diphtheroids
    a. neisseria
    a. streptococcus
analbuminemia
analgesic
    a. nephropathy
    a. neuropathy
anandria
anangioplasia
anaphia
anaphoresis
anaphylactic shock
anaphylactoid
    a. purpura
    a. reaction
anaphylaxis
    generalized a.
    passive a.
anaplasia
Anaplasma
Anaplasmataceae
anaplastic
    a. adenocarcinoma
    a. carcinoma

anaplerotic
anasarca
anasarcous sound
anastalis
Anatrichosoma
Ancylidae
Ancylostoma
    A. braziliense
    A. caninum
    A. duodenale
Anders' disease (adiposis
  tuberosa simplex)
Andersen's
    A's disease
      (amylopectinosis)
    A's syndrome (cystic
      fibrosis of the pancreas)
andreioma
andreoblastoma
androblastoma
androgynoid
andrology
andropathy
anectasis
anemia, anaemia
    achrestic a.
    achylic a.
    acquired sideroachrestic a.
    acute posthemorrhagic a.
    Addison's a.
    Addison-Biermer a.
    anhematopoietic a.
    aplastic a.
    aregenerative a.
    autoimmune hemolytic a.
      (AIHA)
    Bartonella a.
    Biermer's a.

Additional Entries

anemia, anaemia *(continued)*
    Blackfan-Diamond a.
    cameloid a.
    chlorotic a.
    chronic a.
    congenital
        dyserythropoietic a.
    congential hypoplastic a.
    congenital nonspherocytic
        hemolytic a.
    Cooley's a.
    cow's milk a.
    deficiency a.
    Diamond-Blackfan a.
    dilution a.
    dimorphic a.
    drug-induced immune
        hemolytic a.
    dyserythropoietic a.
    elliptocytotic a.
    erythroblastic a. of
        childhood
    essential a.
    Estren-Damashek a.
    familial erythroblastic a.
        (thalassemia)
    familial hemolytic a.
    Fanconi's a.
    folic acid deficiency a.
    glucose-6-phosphate
        dehydrogenase
        deficiency a.
    goat's milk a.
    ground itch a.
    Heinz body hemolytic a.
    hemolytic a.
    hemolytic a., acquired
    hemolytic a., acute

anemia, anaemia *(continued)*
    hemolytic a. congenital
    hemolytic a., congenital
        nonspherocytic
    hemolytic a., hereditary
        nonspherocytic
    hemolytic a., immune
    hemolytic a., infectious
    hemolytic a.,
        microangiopathic
    hemolytic a., toxic
    hemorrhagic a.
    hypochromic a.
    hypochromic a.,
        idiopathic
    hypochromic microcytic a.
    a. hypochromica
        siderochrestica
        hereditaria
    hypoplastic a.
    hypoplastic a., congenital
    iatrogenic a.
    idiopathic a.
    intertropical a.
    iron deficiency a.
    leukoerythroblastic a.
    macrocytic a.
    macrocytic a., nutritional
    macrocytic a., tropical
    Mediterranean a.
    megaloblastic a.
    megaloblastic a., familial
    megalocytic a.
    microangiopathic a.
    microcytic a.
    microdrepanocytic a.
    miner's a.
    mountain a.

Additional Entries

anemia, anaemia *(continued)*
- myelophthisic a.
- a. neonatorum
- normochromic a.
- normocytic a.
- nosocomial a.
- nutritional a.
- osteosclerotic a.
- pernicious a.
- pernicious a., juvenile
- phenylhydrazine a.
- physiologic a.
- polar a.
- posthemorrhagic a., acute
- posthemorrhagic a., of newborn
- primaquine-sensitive a.
- protein deficiency a.
- a. pseudoleukemica infantum
- pure red cell a.
- pyridoxine-responsive a.
- a. refractoria sideroblastica
- refractory a.
- refractory sideroblastic a.
- scorbutic a.
- sickle cell a.
- sideroachrestic a.
- sideroblastic a.
- sideropenic a.
- spherocytic a.
- splenic a.
- spur-cell a.
- thrombopenic a.
- tropical a.
- vitamin deficiency a.
- Von Jaksch'a a.

anemic, anaemic
- a. murmur
- a. necrosis

anenzymia
anepiploic
anepithymia
anerethisia
anerythroplasia
ancrythroplastic
anerythropoiesis
anesthekinesis
anesthesia
- angioplastic a.
- cerebral a.
- compression a.
- dissociated a.
- facial a.
- gauntlet a.
- gustatory a.
- hysterical a.
- mental a.
- olfactory a. (anosmia)
- peripheral a.
- segmental a.
- tactile a.
- thalamic hyperesthetic a.
- traumatic a.

anesthetic leprosy
anetoderma
- a. erythematosum

aneurysm
- abdominal a.
- ampullary a.
- aortic arch a.
- aortic sinusal a.
- arteriosclerotic a.
- arteriosclerotic thrombosed a.

Additional Entries

_____
_____
_____
_____

aneurysm *(continued)*
- arteriovenous a.
- arteriovenous pulmonary a.
- atherosclerotic a.
- axial a.
- axillary a.
- bacterial a.
- berry a.
- brain a. (berry a.)
- cardiac a.
- cirsoid a.
- compound a.
- congenital a.
- congenital cerebral a.
- congenital ruptured a.
- cylindroid a.
- dissecting a.
- ectatic a.
- embolic a.
- endogenous a.
- erosive a.
- exogenous a.
- false a.
- fusiform a.
- hernial a.
- infected a.
- innominate a.
- intracranial a.
- lateral a.
- luetic a.
- miliary a.
- mycotic a.
- orbital a.
- Park's a.
- pelvic a.
- popliteal a.
- Pott's a.

aneurysm *(continued)*
- racemose a.
- Rasmussen's a.
- Richet's a.
- Rodrigues' a.
- ruptured a.
- saccular a.
- serpentine a.
- Shekelton's a.
- spurious a.
- suprasellar a.
- syphilitic a.
- thoracic a.
- thrombosed a.
- traumatic a.
- true a.
- tubular a.
- varicose a.
- venous a.
- ventricular a.

aneurysmal
- a. bone cyst
- a. dilatation
- a. varix

Angelucci's syndrome

angiectasis

angiitis
- allergic granulomatous a.
- consecutive a.
- leukocytoclastic a.
- necrotizing a.
- visceral a.

angina
- abdominal a.
- a. acuta
- agranulocytic a.
- benign croupous a.
- Bretonneau's a.

Additional Entries

angina *(continued)*
   a. catarrhalis
   a. cordis
   a. cruris
   a. decubitus
   a. dyspeptica
   a. epiglottidea
   exudative a.
   a. follicularis
   a. gangrenosa
   hippocratic a.
   hysteric a.
   intestinal a.
   a. inversa
   lacunar a.
   a. laryngea
   Ludwig's a.
   malignant a.
   a. membanacea
   neutropenic a.
   a. nosocomii
   a. pectoris
   a. pectoris vasomotoria
   a. phlegmonosa
   Plaut's a.
   preinfarction a.
   Prinzmetal's a.
   pseudomembranous a.
   a. rheumatica
   a. scarlatinosa
   Schultz's a.
   a. simplex
   a. sine dolore
   a. tonsillaris
   a. trachealis
   a. ulcerosa
   variant a. pectoris
   vasomotor a.

angina *(continued)*
   Vincent's a.
aginose
anginosis
angioataxia
angioblastic meningioma
angioblastoma
angiocarditis
angiochondroma
angiocrinosis
angiodermatitis
angiodysplasia
angiodystrophia
angioectasia
angioectatic
angioedema
   hereditary a.
   vibratory a.
angioedematous
angioelephantiasis
angioendothelioma
angiofibroblastoma
angiofibroma
   juvenile a.
   nasopharyngeal a.
angioglioma
angiogliomatosis
angiogranuloma
angiohemophilia
angiohyalinosis
   a. hemorrhagica
angioimmunoblastic
   lymphadenopathy
angioinvasive adenoma
angiokeratoma
   a. circumscriptum
   a. corpus diffusum
   a. Fordyce

Additional Entries

angiokeratoma *(continued)*
    a. Mibellia
    a. of scrotum
    solitary a.
angiokeratosis
angioleiomyoma
angioleucitis (lymphangitis)
angiolipoleiomyoma
  (angiomyolipoma)
angiolipoma
angiolith
angiolupoid
angiolymphangioma
angiolymphitis
angioma
    a. arteriale racemosum
    arteriovenous a. of brain
    capillary a.
    a. cavernosum cavernous
    cherry a.
    a. cutis
    fissural a.
    hypertrophic a.
    a. lymphaticum
    plexiform a.
    senile a.
    serpiginosum a.
    simple a.
    spider a.
    telangiectatic a.
    a. venosum racemosum
    venous a. of brain
angiomalacia
angiomatosis
    cerebroretinal a. (von
      Hippel-Lindau disease)
    encephalofacial a.
    encephalotrigeminal a.

angiomatosis *(continued)*
    hepatic a.
    a. of retina
    retinocerebral a.
angiomatous meningioma
angiomegaly
angiomyolipoma
angiomyoma
angiomyopathy
angiomyosarcoma
angiomyxoma
angionecrosis
angioneoplasm
angioneuralgia
angioneuroma
angioneuropathy
angioneurosis
angioneurotic
    a. edema
angionoma
angiopancreatitis
angioparalysis
angioparesis
angiopathology
angiopathy
angiophakomatosis
angioreticuloendothelioma
  (Kaposi's sarcoma)
angioreticuloma
angiorrhexis
angiosarcoma
    a. myxomatodes
angiosclerosis
angiosclerotic
angioscotoma
angiospasm
angiospastic
angiostenosis

Additional Entries

angiosteosis
angiostrongyliasis
Angiostrongylus
    A. cantonensis
    A. vasorum
angiotelectasis
angiitis (angiitis)
anglicus sudor
angophrasia
angor
    a. animi
    a. ocularis
    a. pectoris
anhidrosis
anhidrotic
anhydremia
anhypnosis
aniacinamidosis
aniacinosis
anincretinosis
anisakiasis
Anisakis
    A. marina
aniseikonia
aniseikonic
anisoaccommodation
anisochromasia
anisochromia
anisocoria
anisocytosis
anisodactylous
anisodactyly
anisohypercytosis
anisokaryosis
anisoleukocytosis
anisomastia
anisomelia
anisometropia

anisonucleolinosis
anisonucleosis
anisophoria
anisopia
anisorhythmia
anisotropic
anisuria
ankyloblepharon
    a. filiforme adnatum
ankylocheilia
ankylocolpos
ankylodactyly
ankyloglossia
    complete a.
    partial a.
    a. superior
ankylosing spondylitis
ankylosis
    artificia a.
    bony a.
    cricoarytenoid joint a.
    extracapsular a.
    false a.
    fibrous a.
    intracapsular a.
    osseous a.
    spurious a.
    stapedial a.
    true a.
ankylostomiasis
ankylotic
ankylurethria
anoia
anomalous
anomaly
    Alder-Reilly a.
    Alder's a.
    Aristotle's a.

Additional Entries

anomaly *(continued)*
    Axenfeld's a.
    Chediak-Higashi a.
    Chediak-Steinbrinck-
      Higashi a.
    chromosomal a.
    congenital a.
    developmental a.
    Ebstein's a.
    Freund's a.
    May-Hegglin a.
    Pelger-Huet nucular a.
    Poland's a.
    Rieger's a.
    Uhl's a.
    Undritz a.
    vascular a.
anonychia
anonymous mycobacterium
Anopheles
    A. maculipennis
anophthalmia
Anoplocephalidae
Anoplura
anorectic
anorectitis
anorexia
    a. nervosa
anorthopia
anosmia
    a. gustatoria
    preferential a.
    a. respiratoria
anosognosia
anosteoplasia
anostosis
anotropia
anoxemia

anoxemic
anoxia
    altitude a.
    anemic a.
anoxic a.
    fulminating a.
    histotoxic a.
    hypoxic a.
    myocardial a.
    neonatorum a.
    stagnant a.
anoxic
    a. encephalopathy
Anoxyphotobacteria
ANS (arteriolonephrosclerosis)
Anthomyia
    A. canicularis
    A. incisura
    A. manicata
    A. salatrix
    A. scalaris
Anthomyiidae
anthraconecrosis
anthracosilicosis
anthracosis
    a. linguae
anthrax
    agricultural a.
    cerebral a.
    cutaneous a.
    gastrointestinal a.
    industrial a.
    inhalational a.
    intestinal a.
    malignant a.
    meningeal a.
    pulmonary a.
    symptomatic a.

Additional Entries

antrodynia
antronalgia
anuresis
anuria
    angioneurotic a.
    calculous a.
    obstructive a.
    postrenal a.
    renal a.
    suppressive a.
anuric
anus
    ectopic a.
    imperforate a.
    preternatural a.
    a. vesicalis
    a. vestibularis
    vulvovaginal a.
anusitis
aortalgia
aortic
    a. aneurysm
    a. arch syndrome
    a. regurgitation
    a. septal defect
    a. stenosis
aortitis
    bacterial a.
    Dohle-Heller a.
    luetic a.
    nummular a.
    rheumatoid a.
    syphilitic a.
aortopathy
aortosclerosis
apallesthesia
apallic syndrome
Apansporoblastina

aparathyreosis
aparathyroidism
aparathyrosis
aparthrosis
apastia
apathism
apathy
apepsia
apepsinia
aperistalsis
Apert's disease (syndrome)
Apert-Crouzon disease
aphagia
aphakia
aphalangia
aphasia
    acoustic a.
    ageusic a.
    amnemonic a.
    amnesic a.
    anomic a.
    anosmic a.
    associative a.
    ataxic a.
    auditory a.
    Broca's a.
    central a.
    combined a.
    commissural a.
    complete a.
    conduction a.
    cortical a.
    expressive a.
    expressive-receptive a.
    fluent a.
    frontocortical a.
    frontolenticular a.
    functional a.

Additional Entries

aphasia *(continued)*
    gibberish a.
    global a.
    graphomotor a.
    Grashey's a.
    impressive a.
    intellectual a.
    jargon a.
    Kussmaul's a.
    lenticular a.
    Lichtheim's a.
    mixed a.
    motor a.
    nominal a.
    nonfluent a.
    optic a.
    parieto-occipital a.
    pathematic a.
    pictorial a.
    psychosensory a.
    receptive a.
    semantic a.
    sensory a.
    subcortical a.
    syntactical a.
    tactile a.
    temporoparietal a.
    total a.
    transcortical a.
    true a.
    verbal a.
    visual a.
    Wernicke's a.
aphemesthesia
aphemia
aphemic
aphonia
    a. clericorum
aphonia *(continued)*
    hysteric a.
    a. paralytica
    spastic a.
aphosphagenic
aphosphorosis
aphotesthesia
aphrasia
aphthae
    Bednar's a.
    contagious a.
    epizootic a.
    Mikulicz's a.
    recurring scarring a.
aphthoid
aphthongia
aphthosis
aphthous
    a. fever
    a. stomatitis
    a. ulceration
aphthovirus
apical
    a. abscess
    a. canaliculi
    a. granuloma
APL (acute promyelocytic leukemia)
aplasia
    a. axialis extracorticalis congenita
    congenital thymic a.
    a. cutis congenita
    erythroid a.
    germinal a.
    gonadal a.
    granulocytic a.
    hematopoietic a.

Additional Entries

aplasia *(continued)*
    hereditary retinal a.
    megakaryocytic a.
    nuclear a.
    a. of ovary
    pure red cell a.
    retinal a.
    thymic a.
    thymic-parathyroid a.
aplasmic
aplastic
    a. anemia
    a. bone marrow
    a. crisis
APN (acute pyelonephritis)
apnea
    deglutition a.
    initial a.
    late a.
    neonatorum a.
    posthyperventilation a.
    sleep a.
    traumatic a.
apneumatosis
apneumia
apneusis
apocenosis
apocrinitis
apogee
apokamnosis
aponeurositis
apophlegmatic
apoplectic
apoplexia
apoplexy
    abdominal a.
    adrenal a.
    asthenic a.

apoplexy *(continued)*
    bulbar a.
    capillary a.
    cerebellar a.
    cerebral a.
    delayed a.
    embolic a.
    fulminating a.
    heat a.
    gravescent a.
    neonatal a.
    ovarian a.
    pancreatic a.
    parturient a.
    pituitary a.
    placental a.
    pontile a.
    Raymond's a.
    renal a.
    spinal a.
    thrombotic a.
    traumatic late a.
    uteroplacental a.
apoptosis
aposia
apositia
apostasis
aposthia
appendagitis
    epiploic a.
appendicitis
    actinomycotic a.
    acute a.
    acute gangrenous a.
    acute suppurative a.
    amebic a.
    catarrhal a.
    chronic a.

Additional Entries

appendicitis *(continued)*
    a. by contiguity
    focal a.
    foreign body a.
    fulminating a.
    gangrenous a.
    a. granulosa
    helminthic a.
    left-sided a.
    lumbar a.
    a. obliterans
    obstructive a.
    perforating a.
    purulent a.
    recurrent a.
    relapsing a.
    segmental a.
    skip a.
    stercoral a.
    subperitoneal a.
    suppurative a.
    traumatic a.
    verminous a.
appendicolithiasis
appendicopathia oxyurica
apraxia
    akinetic a.
    amnestica a.
    Brun's a. of gait
    classic a.
    constructional a.
    cortical a.
    ideational a.
    ideokinetic a.
    ideomotor a.
    innervation a.
    Liepmann's a.
    limb-kinetic a.

apraxia *(continued)*
    motor a.
    sensory a.
    transcortical a.
apraxic
aproctia
aprosopia
apselaphesia
apsithyria
aptyalism
apulmonism
Arachis
    A. hypogaea
Arachnia
    A. propionica
Arachnida
arachnodactyly
    contractural a.
    congenital a.
arachnoidism
arachnoiditis
Aran-Duchenne disease
arborvirus
arbovirus
    Group A
    Group B
    Group C
    Group unclassified
arcus senilis
ARD (acute respiratory disease)
ARDS (acute respiratory distress syndrome)
areflexia
Arenaviridae
arenavirus
ARF (acute renal failure, acute respiratory failure)
Argas

Additional Entries

Argas *(continued)*
    A. persicus
    A. reflexus
Argentinian hemorrhagic fever virus
argininemia
argyria
arhigosis
arhinencephaly
Arias syndrome
ariboflavinosis
Aristotle's anomaly
Arizona
    A. arizonae
    A. hinshawii
Armigeres
    A. obturbans
Armillifer
    A. armillatus
    A. moniliformis
Arnold-Chiari malformation
arrest
    cardiac a.
    deep transverse a.
    developmental a.
    epiphyseal a.
    maturation a.
    sinus a.
    spermatogenic a.
    spermatogenic maturation a.
arrhenoblastoma
arrhinencephaly
arrhythmia
    continuous a.
    juvenile a.
    nodal a.
    perpetual a.

arrhythmia *(continued)*
    phasic a.
    respiratory a.
    sinus a.
arteriectopia
arteriolitis
arteriolonephrosclerosis
arteriopathy
    hypertensive a.
arteriosclerosis
    Monckeberg's a.
    a. obliterans
arteriosclerotic
    a. aneurysm
    a. aortic aneurysm
    a. cardiovascular disease
    a. heart disease
    a. thrombosed aneurysm
arteriovenous
    a. aneurysm
    a. fistula
    a. malformation
arteritis
    giant cell a.
    rheumatic a.
    rheumatoid a.
    temporal a.
arthralgia
    rheumatic a.
    a. saturnina
arthritide
arthritis
    acute a.
    acute gouty a.
    acute rheumatic a.
    acute suppurative a.
    atrophic a.
    bacterial a.

Additional Entries

arthritis *(continued)*
    Bekhterev's a.
    chronic inflammatory a.
    chronic proliferative a.
    chronic villous a.
    climactic a.
    cricoarytenoid a.
    a. deformans
    degenerative a.
    exudative a.
    fungal a.
    gouty a.
    hemophilic a.
    hypertrophic a.
    infectious a.
    juvenile a.
    Lyme's a.
    menopausal a.
    a. mutilans
    mycotic a.
    navicular a.
    neuropathic a.
    a. nodosa
    a. pauperum
    proliferative a.
    psoriatic a.
    rheumatoid a.
    rheumatoid a., juvenile
    rheumatoid a. of spine
    septic a.
    a. sicca
    suppurative a.
    syphilitic a.
    tuberculous a.
    uratic a.
    a. urethritica
    venereal a.
    vertebral a.

arthritis *(continued)*
    viral a.
arthrocele
arthrochalasis
    a. multiplex congenita
arthrochondritis
arthroclasia
Arthroderma
Arthrographis
    A. langeroni
arthrogryposis
    congenital multiple a.
arthrokatadysis
arthrokleisis
arthrolithiasis
arthromeningitis
arthroneuralgia
arthronosos
    a. deformans
arthro-onychodysplasia
arthro-ophthalmopathy
    hereditary progressive a.
arthropathia
    a. ovaripriva
    a. psoriatica
arthropathy
    Charcot's a.
    chondrocalcific a.
    inflammatory a.
    neurogenic a.
    neuropathic a.
    osteopulmonary a.
    psoriatic a.
    static a.
    syphilitic a.
    tabetic a.
arthrophyma
arthrorheumatism

Additional Entries

arthrosclerosis
arthrosis
    a. deformans
arthrosteitis
arthrosynovitis
arthroxerosis
Artyfechinostomum
arytenoiditis
AS (Adams-Stokes disease, arteriosclerosis, atherosclerosis)
As. (astigmatism)
asbestosis
ascariasis
ascarid
ascarides
Ascaridia
    A. galli
    A. lineata
Ascaridoidea
Ascaris
    A. alata
    A. canis
    A. lumbricoides
    A. marginata
    A. megalocephala
    A. mystax
    A. ovis
    A. pneumonitis
    A. suis
    A. suum
    A. vermicularis
ascites
    a. adiposus
    agonal a.
    bile a.
    bloody a.
    chyliform a.

ascites *(continued)*
    exudative a.
    fatty a.
    hemorrhagic a.
    hydremic a.
    milky a.
    a. praecox
    pseudochylous a.
    transudative a.
Ascomycetes
ASCVD (arteriosclerotic cardiovascular disease)
asemasia
asemia
    a. graphica
    a. mimica
    a. verbalis
asialia
asiderosis
ASMI (anteroseptal myocardial infarct)
aspalasoma
aspergilloma
aspergillomycosis
aspergillosis
    aural a.
    bronchopneumonic a.
    pulmonary a.
Aspergillus
    A. amsteloidami
    A. auricularis
    A. barbae
    A. bouffardi
    A. candidus
    A. carneus
    A. clavatus
    A. concentricus
    A. cookei

Additional Entries

Aspergillus *(continued)*
   A. fisherii
   A. flavus
   A. fumigatus
   A. giganteus
   A. glaucus
   A. gliocladium
   A. mucoroides
   A. nidulans
   A. niger
   A. niveus
   A. ochraceus
   A. oryzae
   A. parasiticus
   A. pictor
   A. repens
   A. restrictus
   A. sulphureus
   A. sydowi
   A. terreus
   A. versicolor
aspergillustoxicosis
aspermatism
aspermatogensis
aspermia
asphyxia
   blue a.
   a. carbonica
   a. cyanotica
   fetal a.
   a. livida
   local a.
   neonatorum a.
   a. pallida
   secondary a.
   traumatic a.
   white a.
asphyxiation

aspiration pneumonia
asplenia
   functional a.
asplenic
astasia
asteatosis
Asteroccus
asthenia
   myalgic a.
   neurocirculatory a.
   periodic a.
   tropical anhidrotic a.
asthenocoria
asthenopia
   accommodative a.
   hysterical a.
   muscular a.
   nervous a.
   neurasthenic a.
   retinal a.
   tarsal a.
asthenopic
asthenoxia
asthma
   abdominal a.
   allergic a.
   alveolar a.
   atopic a.
   bacterial a.
   bronchial a.
   bronchitic a.
   cardiac a.
   cat a.
   catarrhal a.
   a. convulsivum
   cotton dust a.
   cutaneous a.
   diisocyanate a.

Additional Entries

asthma *(continued)*
    dust a.
    Elsner's a.
    emphysematous a.
    essential a.
    extrinsic a.
    food a.
    grinders' a.
    Heberden's a.
    horse a.
    humid a.
    infective a.
    intrinsic a.
    isocyanate a.
    Kopp's a.
    Millar's a.
    millers' a.
    miners' a.
    nasal a.
    nervous a.
    pollen a.
    potters' a.
    reflex a.
    Rostan's a.
    sexual a.
    spasmodic a.
    steam-fitters' a.
    stone-strippers' a.
    symptomatic a.
    thymic a.
    true a.
    Wichmann's a.
asthmatic bronchitis
astigmatism
    acquired a.
    a. against the rule
    compound a.
    congenital a.

astigmatism *(continued)*
    corneal a.
    direct a.
    hypermetrophic a., compound
    hyperopic a., simple
    inverse a.
    irregular a.
    lenticular a.
    mixed a.
    myopic a.
    myopic a., compound
    myopic a., simple
    oblique a.
    physiological a.
    regular a.
    a. with the rule
astigmia (astigmatism)
astomia
astrocytoma
    anaplastic a.
    fibrillary a.
    fibrous a.
    gemistocytic a.
    Grades I-IV a.
    pilocytic a.
    piloid a.
    protoplasmic a.
astrocytosis
asynclitism
    anterior a.
    posterior a.
asyndesis
asynechia
asynovia
asyntaxia
    a. dorsalis
atactic

Additional Entries

ataxia
- acute a.
- acute cerebellar a.
- alcoholic a.
- autonomic a.
- central a.
- cerebellar a.
- cerebral a.
- a. cordis
- enzootic a.
- family a. (Friedreich's a.)
- Friedreich's a.
- frontal a.
- hereditary a.
- hereditary spinal a.
- hysterical a.
- intrapsychic a.
- kinetic a.
- labyrinthic a.
- Leyden's a.
- locomotor a.
- Marie's a.
- motor a.
- ocular a.
- Sanger Brown a.
- sensory a.
- spinal a.
- spinocerebellar a.
- a.-telangiectasia
- thermal a.
- truncal a.
- vasomotor a.
- vestibular a.

ataxiamnesic
ataxiaphasia
ataxophemia
ATD (asphyxiating thoracic dystrophy)

atelectasis
- absorption a.
- acquired a.
- compression a.
- congenital a.
- initial a.
- lobar a.
- lobular a.
- a. neonatorum
- obstructive a.
- patchy a.
- primary a.
- relaxation a.
- resorption a.
- secondary a.
- segmental a.

atelectatic
atelencephalia
atelia
ateliotic
atelocardia
atelocephalus
atelocephaly
atelochelia
atelocheiria
ateloglossia
atelognathia
atelomyelia
atelopodia
ateloprosopia
atelorachidia
Atelosaccharomyces
atelostomia
athalposis
athelia
atheroma
atheromatosis
atheromatous

Additional Entries

atheromatous *(continued)*
    a. embolus
    a. plaque
atheronecrosis
atherosclerosis
    a. obliterans
atherosclerotic heart disease
athetosis
    double a.
    double congenital a.
    pupillary a.
athiaminosis
athlete's foot
athyroidosis (hypothyroidism)
ATN (acute tubular necrosis)
atocia
atony
atopic
    a. dermatitis
    a. keratoconjunctivitis
atopy
atransferrinemia
Atrax
    A. robustus
atresia
    anal a.
    aortic a.
    aural a.
    biliary a.
    choanal a.
    congenital a.
    duodenal a.
    esophageal a.
    follicular a.
    intestinal a.
    a. iridis
    mitral a.
    prepyloric a.

atresia *(continued)*
    pulmonary a.
    tricuspid a.
    valvular a.
atretocystia
atretogastria
atretolemia
atretometria
atretorrhinia
atretostomia
atreturethria
atrial
    a. anomalous bands
    a. arrhythmia
    a. fibrillation
    a. flutter
    a. premature beat
    a. premature contraction
    a. premature depolarization
    a. septal defect
atrichosis (alopecia)
atriomegaly
atrioventricular block
atrioventricularis communis
atrophedema
atrophia
    a. bulborum hereditaria
    a. cerebri senilis simplex
    a. choroideae et retinae
    a. cutis
    a. cutis senilis
    a. dolorosa
    a. maculosa
    a. maculosa varioliformis cutis
    a. musculorum lipomatosa
    a. senilis

Additional Entries

atrophia *(continued)*
    a. testiculi
atrophic
    a. arthritis
    a. chronic gastritis
    a. endometrium
    a. fenestration
    a. gastritis
    a. glossitis
    a. lichen planus
    a. rhinitis
atrophie
    a. blanche
    a. noir
atrophied
atrophoderma
    a. biotripticum
    idiopathic a. of Pasini and Pierini
    a. maculatum
    a. neuriticum
    a. reticulatum symmetricum faciei
    a. senile
    a. vermicularis
atrophodermatosis
atrophodermia
    a. vermiculata
atrophy
    acquired a.
    acute yellow a.
    Aran-Duchenne muscular a.
    arthritic a.
    black a.
    blue a.
    bone a.
    brown a.

atrophy *(continued)*
    Charcot-Marie a.
    Charcot-Marie-Tooth a.
    circumscribed cerebral a.
    compensatory a.
    compression a.
    concentric a.
    convolutional a.
    correlated a.
    corticostriatospinal a.
    Cruveilhier's a.
    cystic a.
    degenerative a.
    Dejerine-Sottas type of a.
    Dejerine-Thomas a.
    denervated muscle a.
    a. of disuse
    Duchenne-Aran muscular a.
    eccentric a.
    Eichhorst's a.
    endocrine a.
    endometrial a.
    Erb's a.
    essential a.
    exhaustion a.
    facial a.
    facioscapulohumeral muscular a.
    fatty a.
    Fazio-Londe a.
    focal a.
    gastric a.
    granular a. of kidney
    gray a.
    gyrate a. of choroid and retina
    healed yellow a.

Additional Entries

atrophy *(continued)*
    hemifacial a.
    hemilingual a.
    Hoffmann's a.
    Hunt's a.
    idopathic muscular a.
    infantile a.
    inflammatory a.
    interstitial a.
    a. of iris, essential
    ischemic muscular a.
    juvenile muscular a.
    lactation a.
    Landouzy-Dejerine a.
    leaping a.
    Leber's optic a.
    linear a.
    lobar a.
    macular a.
    marantic a.
    mucinous a.
    muscular a.
    muscular a., hypertrophic polyneuritic type
    myelopathic muscular a.
    myopathic a.
    neural a.
    neuritic muscular a.
    neuropathic a.
    neurotic a.
    neurotrophic a.
    numeric a.
    olivocerebellar a.
    olivopontocerebellar a.
    optic a.
    optic a., primary
    optic a., secondary
    pallidal a.

atrophy *(continued)*
    Parrot's a. of newborn
    pathologic a.
    periodontal a.
    peroneal a.
    physiologic a.
    pigmentary a.
    postmenopausal a.
    post traumatic a. of bone
    pressure a.
    progressive choroidal a.
    progressive muscular a.
    progressive neuromuscular a.
    progressive neuropathic (peroneal) muscular a.
    progressive spinal muscular a.
    progressive unilateral facial a.
    pseudohypertrophic muscular a.
    pulp a.
    red a.
    reversionary a.
    rheumatic a.
    segmental dissoriation with brachial muscular a.
    senile a.
    senile a. of skin
    serous a.
    simple a.
    spinal muscular a.
    subacute a. of liver
    subchronic a. of liver
    Sudeck's a.
    Tooth's a.

Additional Entries

atrophy *(continued)*
    traction a.
    traumatic a.
    trophoneurotic a.
    unilateral facial a.
    Vulpian's a.
    Werdnig-Hoffmann a.
    Werdnig-Hoffmann spinal muscular a.
    white a.
    yellow a.
    Zimmerlin's a.
attack
    Adams-Stokes a.
    anxiety a.
    panic a.
    transient ischemic a. (TIA)
    vagal a.
    vasovagal a.
atticitis
atypia
    koilocytotic a.
atypical
    a. hyperplasia
    a. lymphocytes
    a. mycobacterium
    a. pneumonia
    a. primary pneumonia
    a. verrucous endocarditis
Auchmeromyia
    A. luteola
Aujesxky's disease
aura
    a. asthmatica
    auditory a.
    electric a.
    epigastric a.
    epileptic a.

aura *(continued)*
    a. hysterica
    intellectual a.
    kinesthetic a.
    motor a.
    a. procursiva
Aurococcus
Austin-Flint murmur
Australorbis
    A. glabratus
autemesia
autism
    akinetic a.
    early infantile a.
    infantile a.
autoimmune
    a. hemolytic anemia
    a. leukopenia
    a. pancytopenia
    a. thrombocytopenic purpura
    a. thyroiditis
Avellis's syndrome
Axenfeld's anomaly, syndrome
axonapraxia
axonotmesis
Ayerxa's disease, syndrome
Azomonas
Azorean disease
Azospirillum
azotemia
    chloropenic a.
    extrarenal a.
    hypochloremic a.
    postrenal a.
    prerenal a.
    renal a.
azotemic

Additional Entries

azotenesis
azothermia
Azotobacter
Azotobacteraceae

azotorrhea
azoturia
azoturic
azurophilia

Additional Entries

B

Baastrup's disease
Babesia
    B. Microti
babesiosis
Babinski's syndrome
Babinski-Froehlich disease
  (adiposogenital dystrophy)
Bacillaceae
bacillary
    b. dysentery
bacillemia
bacilluria
Bacillus
    B. acidi lactici
    B. aerogenes capsulatus
    B. aertrycke
    B. alvei
    B. ambiguus
    B. anthracis
    B. botulinus
    B. brevis
    B. bronchisepticus
    B. cereus
    B. circulans
    B. coli
    B. diptheriae
    B. dysenteriae
    B. enteritidis
    B. faecalis alcaligenes
    B. fusiformis
    B. influenzae
    B. larvae
    B. leprae
    B. licheniformis
    B. mallei

Bacillus *(continued)*
    B. megatherium
    B. necrophorus
    B. oedematiens
    B. oedematis maligni No. II
    B. pertussis
    B. pestis
    B. pneumoniae
    B. polymyxa
    B. proteus
    B. pseudomallei
    B. pumilus
    B. pyocyaneus
    B. sphaericus
    B. stearothermophilus
    B. subtilis
    B. suipestifer
    B. tetani
    B. tuberculosis
    B. tularense
    B. typhi
    B. typhosus
    B. welchii
    B. whitmori
bacillus
    b. abortivus equinus
    anthrax b.
    Bang's b.
    Battey bacilli
    Boas-Oppler b.
    Bordet-Gengou b.
    butter b.
    Calmette-Guerin b.
    Chauveau's b.

Additional Entries

bacillus *(continued)*
    coliform b.
    colon b.
    diphtheria b.
    Doderlein's b.
    Ducrey's b.
    dysentery bacilli
    enteric b.
    Escherich's b.
    Fick's b.
    Flexner's b.
    Flexner-Strong b.
    Friedlander's b.
    fusiform b.
    Gartner's b.
    Ghon-Sachs b.
    glanders b.
    Hansen's b.
    Hofmann's b.
    hog cholera b.
    Johne's b.
    Klebs-Loffler b.
    Klein's b.
    Koch's b.
    Koch-Weeks b.
    lepra b.
    leprosy b.
    Morax-Axenfeld b.
    Morgan's b.
    Newcastle-Manchester b.
    Nocard's b.
    paracolon bacilli
    Pfeiffer's b.
    plague b.
    Preisz-Nocard b.
    pseudotuberculosis b.
    rhinoscleroma b.
    Schmitz's b.

bacillus *(continued)*
    Schmorl's b.
    Shiga b.
    smegma b.
    Sonne-Duval b.
    Stanley b.
    Strong's b.
    swine rotlauf b.
    tetanus b.
    timothy b.
    tubercle b.
    typhoid b.
    vole b.
    Weeks' b.
    Welch's b.
    Whitmore's b.
backalgia
bacteremia
bacteremic shock
bacteria
    gram-negative b.
    gram-positive b.
    intermediate coliform b.
    monocytogenes b.
bacterial
    b. endaortitis
    b. endocarditis
    b. virus
bacteriemia
Bacterionema
    B. matruchotii
bacteriophytoma
bacteriosis
bacteriospermia
bacteriotoxemia
Bacterium
    B. actinomycetem comitans

Additional Entries

Bacterium *(continued)*
    B. aerogenes
    B. aeruginosum
    B. anitratum
    B. cholerae suis
    B. cloacae
    B. coli
    B. dysenteriae
    B. faecalis alcaligenes
    B. mirabilis
    B. pestis bubonicae
    B. sonnei
    B. subgroup B
    B. tularense
    B. typhosum
bacterium
    acid-fast b.
    aerobic b.
    anaerobic b.
    autotrophic b.
    beaded b.
    bifid b.
    blue-green b.
    Chauveau's b.
    chemoautotrophic b.
    chemoheterotrophic b.
    chromogenic b.
    coliform b.
    coryneform b.
    Dar es Salaam b.
    denitrifying b.
    facultative b.
    gram-negative b.
    gram-positive b.
    hemophilic b.
    heterotrophic b.
    higher bacteria
    hydrogen b.

bacterium *(continued)*
    iron b.
    lysogenic b.
    mesophilic b.
    nitrifying b.
    nodule b.
    nonsulfur b., purple
    organotrophic b.
    parasitic b.
    pathogenic b.
    photoautotrophic b.
    photoheterotrophic b.
    psychrophilic b.
    purple b.
    pyogenic b.
    pyrogenic b.
    rough b.
    saprophytic b.
    smooth b.
    sulfur b.
    sulfur b., purple
    thermophilic b.
    toxigenic b.
    water b.
bacteriuria
bacteriuric
Bacteroidaceae
Bacterioides
    B. asaccharolyticus
    B. bivius
    B. capillosus
    B. clostridiiformis
    B. corrodens
    B. disiens
    B. distasonis
    B. eggerthii
    B. fragilis
    B. funduliformis

Additional Entries

Bacterioides *(continued)*
    B. fusiformis
    B. intermedius
    B. melaninogenicus
    B. nodosus
    B. ochraceus
    B. oralis
    B. ovatus
    B. pneumosintes
    B. praeacutus
    B. putredinis
    B. ruminicola
    B. ruminicola brevis
    B. serpens
    B. splanchnicus
    B. thetaiotaomicron
    B. uniformis
    B. ureolyticus
    B. vulgatus
bacteroides
bacteroidosis
bacteruria
Bactoscilla
baculovirus
Baelz's disease
Baerensprung's erythrasma
Bafverstedt's syndrome
bagassosis
Bahia ulcer
Baker's cyst
balanitis
    amebic b.
    b. circinata
    b. circumscripta plasmacellularis
    b. diabetica
    erosive b.
    Follmann's b.

balanitis *(continued)*
    b. gangraenosa
    gangrenous b.
    phagedenic b.
    plasma cell b.
    b. xerotica obliterans
balanocele
balanochlamyditis
balanoposthitis
    chronic circumscribed plasmocytic b.
    enzootic b.
    specific gangrenous and ulcerative b.
balanoposthomycosis
balanorrhagia
Balanosporida
balantidial
balantidiasis
balantidiosis
Balantidium
    B. coli
    B. suis
balantidosis
baldness
    common male b.
Baller-Gerold syndrome
ballismus
Balme's cough
Bamberger's albuminuria
Bamberger-Marie disease
Bancroft's filariasis
bancroftosis
Bang's
    B. bacillus
    B. disease
Bannister's disease
Banti's disease, syndrome

Additional Entries

baragnosis
Barany's symptom
barbaralalia
Barber's psoriasis
Barbulanympha
Barcoo disease, rot
Bard-Pic syndrome
Bardet-Biedl syndrome
baresthesia
Bargen's streptococcus
baritosis
Barlow's disease, syndrome
barosinusitis
barotitis
    b. media
barotrauma
    otitic b.
    sinus b.
Barraquer's disease
Barre-Guillain syndrome
Barrett's ulcer
Bart's syndrome
Barth's hernia
bartholinitis
Bartholin's
    B. abscess
    B. cyst
Bartonella
    B. bacilliformis
Bartonellaceae
bartonelliasis
bartonellosis
Bartter's syndrome
baruria
baryesthesia
barytosis
basal cell
    b. c. carcinoma

basal cell *(continued)*
    b. c. hyperplasia
    b. c. nevus syndrome
    b. c. papilloma
basaloid carcinoma
basaloma
basedoid
Basedow's disease
basiarachnitis
basiarachnoiditis
Basidiobolus
    B. haptosporus
    B. meristosporus
Basidiomycetes
basket
    Alzheimer's b.
Bassen-Kornzweig syndrome
bathrocephaly
bathyanesthesia
Batten's disease
Battey
    B. bacilli
    B. -type mycobacterium
Baume's symptom
Bayle's disease
Bazin's disease
BB (blue bloaters, breakthrough
    bleeding)
BBB (bundle branch block)
BCE (basal cell epithelioma)
Beard's disease
Bearn-Kunkel-Slater syndrome
Beau's disease, syndrome
beauvariosis
Beauveria
Becker's dystrophy
Becker's nevus

Additional Entries

Beckwith-Wiedemann syndrome
Bednar's apthna
Bedsonia (Chlamydia)
Beggiatoa
Beggiatoaceae
Beggiatoales
begma
Behcet's syndrome
Behier-Hardy sign
Beigel's disease
Bekhterev's arthritis
Belascaris
Bell's
    B. mania
    B. palsy
Bence Jones
    B. J. albumosuria
    B. J. proteinuria
bends
Benedikt's syndrome
Bennett's
    B. disease
    B. fracture
Benson's disease
Berger's
    B. disease
    B. paresthesia
    B. symptom
Bergeron's chorea
beriberi
beriberic
Berlin's disease, edema
Bernard-Horner syndrome
Bernard-Soulier disease
Berhardt's disease
Bernhardt-Roth disease
berry aneurysm

Bertiella
    B. mucronata
    B. studeri
berylliosis
Besnier's prurigo
Besnier-Boeck disease
Besnoitia
    B. bennetti
    B. besnoiti
    B. darlingi
    B. jellisoni
    B. tarandi
Best's disease
Bezold's abscess
Bianchi's syndrome
Biederman's sign
Biedl's disease, syndrome
Bielschowsky-Jansky disease
Biermer's anemia
Biernacki's sign
bifascicular block
Bifidobacterium
    B. adolescentis
    B. bifidum
    B. cornutum
    B. eriksonii
    B. infantis
bigeminy
    nodal b.
    ventricular b.
bile
    b. canaliculi
    b. infarct
    b. nephrosis
    b. stasis
bile duct
    b. d. adenoma
    b. d. canaliculus

Additional Entries

bile duct *(continued)*
    b. d. carcinoma
Bilharzia
bilharziasis
bilharzioma
bilharziosis
biliary
    b. achalasia
    b. atresia
    b. cirrhosis
    b. fistula
    b. obstruction
bilious
biliousness
bilirachia
bilirubin
    b. encephalopathy
bilirubinuria
Billroth's disease
binasal hemianopsia
Binswanger's dementia (encephalitis)
Biomphalaria
    B. glabrata
bird-arm
bird-leg
Birkett's hernia
bisalbuminemia
BJ (Bence Jones)
BL (Burkitt's lymphoma)
Bitot's spots
bituminosis
Bivalvulida
Bjerrum's scotoma
black
    b. fly
    b. hairy tongue
    b. lung disease

Blackfan-Diamond anemia
blackout
bladder
    atonic b.
    atonic neurogenic b.
    automatic b.
    autonomous b.
    fasciculated b.
    irritable b.
    motor paralytic b.
    nervous b.
    neurogenic b.
    paralytic b.
    saculated b.
    sensory paralytic b.
    spastic b.
    uninhibited neurogenic b.
blast
    b. cell leukemia
    b. crisis
Blastobacter
Blastocrithidia
Blastocystitis
    B. hominis
blastoma
    pluricentric b.
    unicentric b.
Blastomyces
    B. brasiliensis
    B. coccidioides
    B. dermatitidis
blastomyces
blastomycosis
    Brazilian b.
    cutaneous b.
    European b.
    keloidal b.
    North American b.

Additional Entries

blastomycosis *(continued)*
    South American b.
    systemic b.
blastophthoria
Blattabacterium
blennadenitis
blennemesis
blennorrhagia
blennorrhagic
blennorrhea
    b. adultorum
    inclusion b.
    b. neonatorum
    Stoerk's b.
blennorrheal
blennothorax
blennuria
blepharadenitis
blepharitis
    b. angularis
    b. ciliaris
    b. marginalis
    nonulcerative b.
    seborrheic b.
    b. squamosa
    squamous seborrheic b.
    b. ulcerosa
blepharoadenitis
blepharoadenoma
blepharoatheromablepharochalasis
blepharochromidrosis
bleparoclonus
blepharoconjunctivitis
Blepharocorynthinia
blepharodiastasis
blepharoncus
blepharopachynis
blepharophimosis

blepharoplegia
blepharoptosis
blepharopyorrhea
blepharospasm
    essential b.
    symptomatic b.
blepharosynechia
Blessig's cysts
blighted ovum
blindness
    amnesic color b.
    blue b.
    blue-yellow b.
    Bright's b.
    color b.
    concussion b.
    cortical b.
    cortical psychic b.
    day b.
    eclipse b.
    electric light b.
    epidemic b.
    flight b.
    functional b.
    legal b.
    letter b.
    mind b.
    moon b.
    night b.
    note b.
    object b.
    psychic b.
    red b.
    red-green b.
    river b.
    snow b.
    soul b.
    syllabic b.

Additional Entries

blindness *(continued)*
    text b.
    total b.
    twilight b.
    word b.
    yellow b.
blister
    blood b.
    fever b.
    Marochetti's b's
    water b.
Bloch-Sulzberger syndrome
block
    adrenergic b.
    alveolar-capillary b.
    arborization b.
    bundle-branch b.
    ear b.
    heart b.
    mental b.
    Mobitz b.
    peri-infarction b.
    sinoatrial b.
    sinus b.
    spinal subarachnoid b.
    ventricular b.
    Wenckebach b.
Blocq's disease
blood
    b. clot
    b. coagulation disorder
    b. dyscrasia
    b. fluke
    b. loss anemia
    b. poisoning
    sludged b.
Bloodgood's disease
Bloom's syndrome

Blount's disease
Blums' syndrome
Blumenthal's disease
blunt duct adenosis
BN (branchial neuritis)
BNO (bladder neck obstruction)
Boas-Oppler bacillus
Bochdalek's hernia
Bockhart's impetigo
Bodo
    B. caudatus
    B. saltans
    B. urinaria
Bodonidae
body (bodies)
    Aschoff's b's
    asteroid b.
    Auer b's
    Bracht-Wachter b's
    brassy b.
    Cabot's ring b's
    Call-Exner b's
    cancer b's
    coccoid x b's
    Councilman b's
    cytoid b's
    foreign b.
    gamma-Favre b.
    Gordon's elementary b.
    Guarnieri's b's
    Halberstaedter-Prowazek b's
    Harting b's
    Hassall-Henle b's
    Heinz b's
    Heinz-Ehrlich b's
    Howell-Jolly b's
    inclusion b's

Additional Entries

body (bodies) *(continued)*
    Lafora's b's
    L.C.L. b's
    Lewy b's
    Lindner's initial b's
    Lipschutz b's
    Marchal b's
    Masson b's
    melon-seed b.
    Michaelis-Gutmann b's
    Mooser b's
    Morner's b.
    Negri b's
    Neill-Mooser b.
    Paschen b's
    Pick b's
    Plimmer's b's
    Prowazek's b's
    psammoma b.
    pyknotic b's
    Reilly b's
    Renaut's b's
    Ross's b's
    Schaumann's b's
    trachoma b's
Boeck's
    B. disease
    B. sarcoid
Boerhaave's syndrome
Bogaert's disease
Boletus
    B. satanas
Bombus californicus
Bonnevie-Ullrich syndrome
Bonnier's syndrome
bony
    b. ankylosis
Book's syndrome

Bordetella
    B. bronchiseptica
    B. parapertussis
    B. pertussis
Bordet-Gengou bacillus
Borna disease
Bornholm disease
Borrelia
    B. aegyptica
    B. anserina
    B. berbera
    B. buccalis
    B. carteri
    B. caucasica
    B. duttonii
    B. hermsii
    B. hispanica
    B. kochii
    B. neotropicalis
    B. novyi
    B. parkeri
    B. perscia
    B. recurrentis
    B. refringens
    B. theileri
    B. turicatae
    B. venezuelensis
    B. vincentii
borreliosis
Borst-Jadassohn intraepidermal basal cell epithelioma
Bostock's catarrh (disease)
bothriocephaliasis
Bothriocephalus
botryoid
    b. rhabdomyosarcoma
    b. sarcoma
botryomycosis

Additional Entries

botryomycotic
botrytimycosis
Botrytis
    B. bassiana
    B. tenella
botulin
botulism
    infant b.
    wound b.
botulismotoxin
Bouchard's disease
Bourneville's disease
boutonneuse fever
Bouveret's disease
Bovimyces pleuropneumoniae
Bowen's disease
Boston exanthem
BPH (benign prostatic hypertrophy)
Br. (Brucella)
brachial
    b. neuritis
brachialgia
    b. statica paresthetica
brachiocyrtosis
Bracht-Wachter lesion
Brachyarcus
brachybasia
brachycardia (bradycardia)
brachycheilia
brachycronic
brachydactyly
brachyesophagus
brachyfacial
brachygnathous
brachymetacarpia
brachymetapody
brachymetatarsia

brachyphalangia
brachyskelous
Bradshaw's albumosuria
bradyacusia
bradyarrhythmia
bradyarthria
bradyauxesis
Bradybaena
bradycardia
    Branham's b.
    cardiomuscular b.
    central b.
    essential b.
    junctional b.
    nodal b.
    postinfective b.
    sinoatrial b.
    sinus b.
    b.-tachycardia syndrome
    vagal b.
bradycardiac
bradydiastole
bradyecoia
bradyesthesia
bradyglossia
bradykinesis
bradykinetic
bradylalia
bradylexia
bradylogia
bradyphagia
bradyphrasia
bradyphrenia
bradypnea
bradyrhythmia
bradysphygmia
bradystalsis
bradytachycardia

Additional Entries

bradytrophia
bradyuria
Braid's strabismus
brain death syndrome
Branhamella
    B. catarrhalis
Branham's sign
breast
    caked b.
    chicken b.
    Cooper's irritable b.
    funnel b.
    pigeon b.
    proemial b.
    shoe-maker's b.
    shotty b.
    thrush b.
    b. tumors
Breda's disease
Breisky's disease
Brennemann's syndrome
Brenner tumor
Bretonneau's angina
Breus mole
Brevibacterium
brevicollis
Brewer's infarcts
bridging
    b. hepatic necrosis
Brieger's cachexia
Bright's blindness
brightic
brightism
Brill's disease
Brill-Symmers disease
Brill-Zinsser disease
Brinton's disease
Brion-Kayser disease

Briquet's syndrome
Brissaud's
    B. dwarf
    B. infantilism
    B. scoliosis
Brissaud-Sicard syndrome
broad
    b.-beta disease
    b. fish tapeworm
Broadbent's sign
Broca's amnesia
Brockenbrough's sign
Brock's syndrome
Brodie's abscess
bromhidrosis
bromidrosis (bromhidrosis)
bronchadenitis
bronchial
    b. adenoma
    b. asthma
    b. carcinoma
bronchiarctia
bronchiectasia
bronchiectasic
bronchiectasis
    capillary b.
    cylindrical b.
    cystic b.
    dry b.
    follicular b.
    fusiform b.
    saccular b.
bronchiectatic
bronchiloquy
bronchiocele
bronchiocrisis
bronchiolar
    b. adenocarcinoma

Additional Entries

bronchiolar *(continued)*
    b. carcinoma
bronchiolectasis
bronchiolitis
    acute obliterating b.
    b. exudativa
    b. fibrosa obliterans
    vesicular b.
bronchiospasm
bronchiostenosis
bronchismus
bronchitis
    acute b.
    acute laryngotracheal b.
    arachidic b.
    asthmatic b.
    capillary b.
    Castellani's b.
    catarrhal b.
    cheesy b.
    chronic b.
    croupous b.
    dry b.
    ether b.
    exudative b.
    fibrinous b.
    hemorrhagic b.
    infectious asthmatic b.
    infectious avian b.
    mechanic b.
    membranous b.
    b. obliterans
    parasitic b.
    phthinoid b.
    plastic b.
    productive b.
    pseudomembranous b.
    putrid b.

bronchitis *(continued)*
    secondary b.
    staphylococcus b.
    streptococcal b.
    suffocative b.
    verminous b.
    vesicular b.
bronchoadenitis
bronchoalveolitis
bronchoaspergillosis
bronchoblastomycosis
bronchoblennorrhea
bronchocandidiasis
bronchocele
bronchoconstriction
bronchodilatation
bronchogenic
    b. carcinoma
    b. cyst
broncholith
broncholithiasis
bronchomalacia
bronchomoniliasis
bronchomycosis
bronchonocardiosis
bronchopathy
bronchoplegia
bronchopleuropneumonia
bronchopneumonia
    acute b.
    acute hemorrhagic b.
    confluent b.
    diffuse b.
    focal b.
    hemorrhagic b.
    necrotizing b.
    sequestration b.
    subacute b.

Additional Entries

bronchopneumonia *(continued)*
    virus b.
bronchopneumonitis
bronchopneumopathy
bronchorrhagia
bronchorrhea
bronchosinusitis
bronchospasm
bronchospirochetosis
bronchostaxis
bronchostenosis
Brooke's
    B. disease
    B. tumor
brown
    b. atrophy
    b. tumor
Brown-Sequard's paralysis
Brucella
    B. abortus
    B. bronchiseptica
    B. canis
    B. melitensis
    B. suis
    B. tularensis
brucella
Brucellaceae
brucellosis
Bruck's disease
Brudzinski's sign
Brugia
    B. malayi
    B. microfilariae
    B. pahangi
bruise
    stone b.
bruit
    aneurysmal b.

bruit *(continued)*
    b. d'airain
    b. de bois
    b. de canon
    b. de choc
    b. de clapotement
    b. de claquement
    b. de craquement
    b. de cuir neuf
    b. de diable
    b. de galop
    b. de grelot
    b. de Leudet
    b. de lime
    b. de moulin
    b. de parchemin
    b. de piaulement
    b. de pot fele
    b. de rape
    b. de rappel
    b. de Roger
    b. de scie
    b. de soufflet
    b. de tabourka
    b. de tambour
    false b.
    Leudet's b.
    b. placentaire
    Roger's b.
    b. skodique
    systolic b.
    Verstraeten's b.
Brunhilde virus
Bruns' disease, syndrome
Brunsting's syndrome
Bruton's
    B. agammaglobulinemia
    B. disease

Additional Entries

brux
bruxism
 centric b.
BT (bladder tumor, brain tumor)
BTB (breakthrough bleeding)
bubonic plague
bubonocele
bubonulus
buccoglossopharyngitis
 b. sicca
Budd's cirrhosis
Budd-Chiari syndrome
Buerger's disease
Buhl's disease
bulbar
 b. conjunctiva
 b. palsy
bulbitis
bulimia
Bulimus
 B. fuchsianus
 B. leachii
Bulinus
Bullis fever
bullosis
 b. diabeticorum
bullous
 b. emphysema
 b. inflammation
 b. lichen planus
 b. pemphigoid
bundle branch block
bunion
bunionette
Bunyamwera virus
Bunyaviridae
bunyavirus
buphthalmos

Burghart's symptom
Burkitt's tumor
burn
 brush b.
 chemical b.
 contact b.
 electric b.
 first-degree b.
 flash b.
 fourth-degree b.
 friction b.
 radiation b.
 second-degree b.
 sun b.
 thermal b.
 third-degree b.
 ultraviolet b.
Burnett's syndrome
bursitis
 Achilles b.
 adhesive b.
 calcific b.
 Duplay's b.
 ischiogluteal b.
 olecranon b.
 omental b.
 pharyngeal b.
 popliteal b.
 prepatellar b.
 radiohumeral b.
 retrocalcaneal b.
 scapulohumeral b.
 subacromial b.
 subdeltoid b.
 superficial calcaneal b.
 Thornwaldt's b.
bursolith
bursopathy

Additional Entries

Buschke's disease, scleredema
Buschke-Lowenstein giant
 condyloma
Buschke-Ollendorff syndrome
Busquet's disease

Busse-Buschke disease
Busse's saccharomyces
Buttiauxella
byssinosis
byssinotic

Additional Entries

C

C. (Clostridium)
C. (Cryptococcus)
CA (carcinoma)
Cacchi-Ricci disease
Cache Valley virus
cachectic
cachexia
    cancerous c.
    c. exophthalmica
    fluoric c.
    hypophyseal c.
    c. hypophysiopriva
    lymphatic c.
    malarial c.
    c. mercurialis
    saturnine c.
    c. strumipriva
    c. suprarenalis
    thyroid c.
    uremic c.
    verminous c.
cacomelia
cacotrophy
CAD (coronary artery disease)
cadmiosis
Caedibacter
caffeinism
Caffey's disease
Caffey-Silverman syndrome
CAG (chronic atrophic gastritis)
CAH (chronic active hepatitis)
CAHD (coronary atherosclerotic heart disease)
caisson disease
calcaneitis
calcaneoapophysitis
calcaneodynia
calcemia
calcibilia
calcicosilicosis
calcicosis
calcific
    c. aortic stenosis
    c. nodular stenosis
    c. stenosis
calcification
    dystrophic c.
    focal c.
    medial c.
    metastatic c.
    Monckeberg's medial c.
calcified
    c. granuloma
    c. granulomatous inflammation
calcifying
    c. ameloblastoma
    c. epithelial odontogenic tumor
    Malherbe's c. epithelioma
calcinosis
    c. circumscripta
    c. cutis
    c. interstitialis
    c. intervertebralis
    tumoral c.
    c. universalis
calciorrhachia
calciotropism
calcipenia

Additional Entries

calcipenic
calcipexy
calciphilia
calciphylaxis
   systemic c.
   topical c.
calcipriva
calciprivic
calcipyelitis
calciuria
calcivirus
calculi
calculosis
calculous
calculus
   alternating c.
   alvine c.
   articular c.
   biliary calculi
   bronchial c.
   calcium oxalate c.
   cholesterol c.
   combination c.
   cystine c.
   decubitus c.
   dental c.
   encysted c.
   fibrin c.
   fusible c.
   gastric c.
   gonecystic c.
   hemic c.
   hemp seed c.
   hepatic c.
   indigo c.
   intestinal c.
   joint c.
   lacrimal c.

calculus *(continued)*
   lacteal c.
   lung c.
   mammary c.
   matrix c.
   metabolic c.
   mulberry c.
   nasal c.
   nephritic c.
   ovarian c.
   oxalate c.
   pancreatic c.
   phosphate c.
   pocketed c.
   preputial c.
   prostatic c.
   renal c.
   renal c., primary
   renal c., secondary
   salivary c.
   serumal c.
   shellac c.
   spermatic c.
   staghorn c.
   stomachic c.
   struvite c.
   subgingival c.
   submorphous c.
   supragingival c.
   tonsillar c.
   urate c.
   urethral c.
   uric acid c.
   urinary c.
   urostealith c.
   uterine c.
   vesical c.
   vesicoprostatic c.

Additional Entries

calculus *(continued)*
    xanthic c.
calicectasis
calicivirus
caliectasis
California encephalitis
    C. e. virus
Calliphora
    C. vomitoria
Calliphoridae
callus
    bony c.
    central c.
    definitive c.
    ensheathing c.
    external c.
    inner c.
    intermediate c.
    medullary c.
    myelogenous c.
    permanent c.
    provisional c.
Calmette-Guerin bacillus
calor
    c. febrilis
    c. fervens
    c. innatus
    c. mordicans
Calvatia
    C. gigantea
Calve-Perthes disease
Calymmatobacterium
    C. donovania
    C. granulomatis
Camurati-Engelmann disease
camphorism
camptocormia
camptodactylia

camptodactylism
camptodactyly
camptomelia
camptomelic
camptospasm
Campylobacter
    C. cinaedi
    C. coli
    C. fecalis
    C. fennilliae
    C. fetus
    C. fetus intestinalis
    C. fetus jejuni
    C. fetus veneralis
    C. pylorus
    C. sputorum
    C. sputorum bubulus
    C. sputorum mucosalis
    C. sputorum sputorum
campylobacteriosis
Canada-Chronkhite syndrome
Canavan's disease
cancer
    acinar c.
    adenoid c.
    c. a deux
    alveolar c.
    aniline c.
    apinoid c.
    areolar c.
    c. atrophicans
    betel c.
    black c.
    boring c.
    branchiogenous c.
    Butter's c.
    buyo cheek c.
    cellular c.

Additional Entries

cancer *(continued)*
    cerebriform c.
    chimney-sweeps' c.
    chondroid c.
    claypipe c.
    colloid c.
    contact c.
    corset c.
    cystic c.
    dendritic c.
    dermoid c.
    duct c.
    dye workers' c.
    encephaloid c.
    c. en cuirasse
    endothelial c.
    epidermal c.
    epithelial c.
    fungous c.
    glandular c.
    green c.
    hard c.
    hematoid c.
    jacket c.
    kang c.
    latent c.
    medullary c.
    melanotic c.
    mule-spinners' c.
    occult c.
    paraffin c.
    pitch-workers' c.
    retrograde c.
    rodent c.
    roentgenologist's
    scirrhous c.
    soft c.
    solanoid c.

cancer *(continued)*
    spindle cell c.
    tar c.
    tubular c.
    villous duct c.
canceremia
cancerigenic
cancerous
cancer-ulcer
cancriform
cancroid
cancrum
    c. nasi
    c. oris
    c. pudendi
Candida
    C. albicans
    C. albidus
    C. guilliermondi
    C. intertrigo
    C. krusei
    C. laurentii
    C. lusitaniae
    C. luteolus
    C. mesenterica
    C. parakrusei
    C. parapsilosis
    C. pseudotropicalis
    C. stellatoidea
    C. tropicalis
    C. vini
    C. viswanathii
candidemia
candidiasis
    cutaneous c.
    endocardial c.
candidid
candidosis

Additional Entries

candiduria
canker sore
canthariasis
cantharidism
Cantharis
    C. vesicatoria
canthitis
CAO (chronic airway obstruction)
Capdepont's disease
Capgras' syndrome
Capillaria
    C. contorta
    C. hepatica
    C. philippinensis
capillariasis
capillaritis
capillaropathy
capistration
Caplan's syndrome
Capnocytophaga
Capripoxvirus
capsitis
capsulitis
    adhesive c.
    hepatic c.
capsuloma
carbohemia
carboluria
carbonemia
carbonuria
    dysoxidative c.
carbuncle
    malignant c.
    renal c.
carbuncular
carbunculoid
carbunculosis

carcinelcosis
carcinemia
carcinogen
carcinogenesis
carcinoid
    c. heart disease
    c. syndrome
    c. tumor
carcinoma
    acinar c.
    adenocystic c.
    adenoid cystic c.
    c. adenomatosum
    adenosquamous c.
    adnexal c.
    adrenal cortical c.
    alveolar c.
    anaplastic c.
    basal cell c.
    basaloid c.
    basosquamous c.
    bile duct c.
    bile duct c., hepatocellular
    bronchial c.
    bronchiolar c.
    bronchogenic c.
    cerebriform c.
    ceruminous c.
    cholangiocellular c.
    chorionic c.
    cloacogenic c.
    colloid c.
    comedo c.
    corpus c.
    cribiform c.
    c. en cuirasse
    c. cutaneum
    cylindrical cell c.

Additional Entries

carcinoma *(continued)*
    duct cell c.
    embryonal c.
    epidermoid c.
    c. epitheliale adenoides
    c. fibrosum
    follicular c.
    gelatiniform c.
    gelatinous c.
    giant cell c.
    c. gigantocellulare
    glandular c.
    granulosa cell c.
    hair matrix c.
    hepatocellular c.
    Hurthle cell c.
    hypernephroid c.
    infantile embryonal c.
    infiltrating duct c.
    infiltrating lobular c.
    inflammatory c.
    c. in situ
    intraductal c.
    intraepidermal c.
    intraepithelial c.
    islet c.
    Krompecher's c.
    Kulchitzky-cell c.
    large cell c.
    lenticular c.
    liver cell c.
    lobular c.
    lymphoepithelial c.
    medullary c.
    melanotic c.
    mesometanephric c.
    metastatic c.
    mixed hepatocellular c.

carcinoma *(continued)*
    c. molle
    mucinous c.
    c. muciparum
    c. mucocellulare
    mucoepidermoid c.
    c. mucosum
    c. myxomatodes
    nasopharyngeal c.
    oat cell c.
    c. ossificans
    papillary c.
    papillary transitional cell c.
    periportal c.
    pleomorphic c.
    preinvasive c.
    prickle cell c.
    recurrent c.
    renal cell c.
    reserve cell c.
    residual c.
    schneiderian c.
    scirrhous c.
    c. scroti
    sebaceous c.
    secondary c.
    signet ring c.
    simplex c.
    small cell c.
    solid c.
    spheroidal cell c.
    spindle cell c.
    c. spongiosum
    squamous cell c.
    string cell c.
    superficial multicentric basal cell c.

Additional Entries

carcinoma *(continued)*
    sweat gland c.
    c. telangiectaticum
    thymic c.
    trabecular c.
    transitional cell c.
    c. tuberosum
    undifferentiated c.
    verrucous c.
    c. villosum
    wolffian duct c.
carcinomata
carcinomatoid
carcinomatosis
carcinomatous
carcinosarcoma
    embryonal c.
carcinosis
    miliary c.
    c. pleurae
    pulmonary c.
carcinous
Cardarelli's sign
cardiac
    c. arrest
    c. cirrhosis
    c. decompensation
    c. edema
    c. enlargement
    c. failure
    c. fibrillation
    c. murmur
    c. sclerosis
    c. standstill
    c. tamponade
    c. valvular malformation
    c. valvular regurgitation
cardiasthenia
cardiasthma
cardiataxia
cardiectasis
Cardiobacterium
    C. hominis
cardiocele
cardiochalasia
cardiocirrhosis
cardiodiosis
cardiodynia
cardiohepatomegaly
cardiomalacia
cardiomegalia
    c. glycogenica
        circumscripta
    c. glycogenica diffusa
cardiomegaly
    glycogenic c.
cardiomelanosis
cardiomyoliposis
cardiomyopathy
    alcoholic c.
    congestive c.
    infiltrative c.
    peripartum c.
    postpartum c.
    primary c.
    restrictive c.
    secondary c.
cardionecrosis
cardioneurosis
cardiopaludism
cardiopath
cardiopathic
    infarctoid c.
cardiopathy
cardiopericarditis
cardiophrenia

Additional Entries

cardioptosia
cardioptosis
cardiorrhexis
cardiosclerosis
cardiospasm
cardiothyrotoxicosis
cardiotoxic
cardiovalvulitis
cardiovascular
    c. malformation
    c. murmur
cardiovascular disease
    arteriosclerotic c. d.
    hypertensive c. d.
cardiovirus
carditis
    rheumatic c.
    streptococcal c.
    verrucous c.
caries
    backward c.
    cemental c.
    central c.
    dental c.
    dental c., primary
    dental c., secondary
    dentinal c.
    dry c.
    enamel c.
    c. fungosa
    internal c.
    lateral c.
    necrotic c.
    pit c.
    c. sicca
    spinal c.
cariogenesis
carnosinase deficiency

carnosinemia
carnosinuria
Caroli's disease
carotenemia
carotenoderma
carotenodermia
carotenosis
carotic
carotid
    c. body tumor
    c. sinus syncope
    c. sinus syndrome
Carpenter's syndrome
carpitis
Carpoglyphus
    C. passularum
carpoptosis
Carrion's disease
cartilaginous
    c. exostosis
    c. metaplasia
Carvallo sign
case
    borderline c.
    index c.
    trial c.
caseating
    c. granuloma
    c. granulomatous inflammation
    c. inflammation
caseation
caseous
    c. inflammation
    c. necrosis
caseworm
Castellanella
    C. castellani

Additional Entries

Castellani's bronchitis
Castellani-Low symptom
catabasis
catacrotic
catacrotism
catadicrotism
catalepsy
cataleptic
cataphasia
cataphoria
cataphylaxis
cataplasia
cataplectic
cataplexy
cataract
    after-c.
    aminoaciduria c.
    atopic c.
    axial fusiform c.
    black c.
    blue dot c.
    brown c.
    calcareous c.
    capsular c.
    cerulean c.
    complete c.
    complicated c.
    congenital c.
    contusion c.
    coralliform c.
    coronary c.
    cortical c.
    cuneiform c.
    cupuliform c.
    dermatogenic c.
    developmental c.
    diabetic c.
    duplication c.

cataract *(continued)*
    electric c.
    embryonal nuclear c.
    embryopathic c.
    evolutionary c.
    galactosemic c.
    glassblower's c.
    glaucomatous c.
    heat c.
    heterochromic c.
    hypermature c.
    hypocalcemic c.
    immature c.
    incipient c.
    intumescent c.
    juvenile c.
    lamellar c.
    mature c.
    membranous c.
    metabolic c.
    morgagnian c.
    nuclear c.
    nutritional deficiency c,
    overripe c.
    polar c.
    postinflammatory c.
    c's of prematurity
    presenile c.
    primary c.
    punctate c.
    pyramidal c.
    radiation c.
    ringform congenital c.
    ripe c.
    rubella c.
    secondary c.
    senile c.
    senile nuclear sclerotic c.

Additional Entries

cataract *(continued)*
- snowflake c.
- Soemmering's ring c.
- spindle c.
- subcapsular c.
- sunflower c.
- supranuclear c.
- sutural c.
- syndermatotic c.
- thermal c.
- total c.
- toxic c.
- traumatic c.
- zonular c.

cataracta
- c. brunescens
- c. caerulea
- c. centralis pulverulenta
- c. complicata
- c. nigra

catarrh
- atrophic c.
- autumnal c.
- Bostock's c.
- hypertrophic c.
- Laennec's c.
- postnasal c.
- sinus c.
- suffocative c.
- vernal c.

catarrhal
- c. appendicitis
- c. conjunctivitis
- c. inflammation

Catarrhina
catatonia
catatonic
- c. schizophrenia

catatricrotic
catatricrotism
cat-bite fever
cat-cry syndrome
Catenabacterium
catheresis
cathexis
cat liver fluke
cat-scratch fever
cauliflower ear
Caulobacter
caumesthesia
causalgia
cause
- constitutional c.
- exciting c.
- immediate c.
- local c.
- precipitating c.
- predisposing c.
- primary c.
- proximate c.
- remote c.
- secondary c.
- specific c.
- ultimate c.

caustic
CAV (congenital absence of vagina)
Cavare's disease
cavernitis
- fibrous c.

cavernositis
cavernous hemangioma
cavitis
Cazenave's disease
CB (chronic bronchitis)

Additional Entries

CBA (chronic bronchitis with asthma)
CBS (chronic brain syndrome)
CCF (congestive cardiac failure)
CCP (ciliocytophthoria)
CDC (Centers for Disease Control)
ceasmic
cebocephalus
cebocephaly
cecitis
cecocele
CEEV (Central European encephalitis virus)
celiac
    c. disease
celioma
celiomyositis
celiopathy
celitis
Cellfalcicula
cellulitis
    anaerobic c.
    clostridial anaerobic c.
    dissecting c. of scalp
    facial c.
    finger c.
    gangrenous c.
    indurated c.
    necrotizing c.
    nonclostridial anaerobic c.
    orbital c.
    pelvic c.
    periurethral c.
    phlegmonous c.
    streptococcal c.
    ulcerative c.
Cellumonas
celluloneuritis
    acute anterior c.
cellulotoxic
Cellvibrio
    C. fulvus
    C. ochraceus
    C. vulgaris
celophlebitis
celoschisis
celosomia
celosomus
celothelioma
celovirus
cementifying fibroma
cementitis
cementoblastoma
cementoma
cementopathia
cementoperiostitis
cementosis
cenadelphus
cenencephalocele
cenesthesiopathy
cenosis
Centers for Disease Control
central
    c. core disease
    c. hemorrhagic necrosis
    c. necrosis
Central European encephalitis virus
centrilobular
    c. emphysema
    c. necrosis
Centrohelida
centronuclear
    c. myopathy
centrosclerosis

Additional Entries

_____
_____
_____
_____

Centruroides
cenurosis
cephalagia
    histamine c.
    pharyngotympanic c.
    quadrantal c.
cephaledema
cephalematocele
cephalgia
cephalhematoma
cephalhydrocele
    c. traumatica
cephalitis
cephalocele
    orbital c.
cephalocyst
cephalodactyly
cephalodiprosopus
cephalodymia
cephalodymus
cephalodynia
cephalohematocele
cephalohematoma
cephaloma
cephalomelus
cephalomania
cephalonia
cephalopathy
cephaloplegia
Cephalopoda
cephalosporiosis
Cephalosporium
    C. falciforme
    C. granulomatis
cephalothoracopagus
    c. disymmetros
    c. monosymmetros
Ceratiomyxa
Ceratium
Ceratophyllus
    C. acutus
    C. fasciatus
    C. gallinae
    C. idahoensis
    C. montanus
    C. punjabensis
    C. silantiewi
    C. tesquorum
Ceratopogonidae
cercaria
cercarial dermatitis
cercocystitis
cercoid
Cercomonas
Cercosphaera addisoni
Cercospora apii
Cercosporalla vexans
cercosporamycosis
cerea flexibilitas
cerebellar
    c. ataxia, familial
    c. ataxia, hereditary
    c. dyssynergia
    c. sarcoma
cerebral
    c. artery stenosis
    c. atrophy
    c. edema
    c. hemorrhage
    c. herniation
    c. infarct
    c. palsy
    c. thrombosis
    c. vascular accident
cerebritis
    saturnine c.

Additional Entries

cerebroma
cerebromalacia
cerebromeningitis
cerebropathia
   c. psychica toxemica
cerebropathy
cerebrosclerosis
cerebrosidosis
cerebrosis
cerebrospinal meningitis
cerebrotendinous
   c. xanthomatosis
cerebrovascular
   c. accident
Cerithidia
   C. cingulata
ceroid
   c. storage disease
ceroma
cerumen
   impacted c.
   inspissated c.
ceruminoma
ceruminosis
ceruminous
   c. adenoma
   c. carcinoma
cervical
   c. intraepithelial neoplasia
   c. polyp
   c. rib syndrome
cervicitis
   granulomatous c.
   traumatic c.
cervicobrachialgia
cervicocolpitis
   c. emphysematosa
cervicodynia
cervicovaginitis
cervix
   incompetent c.
Cestan-Chenais syndrome
Cestan-Raymond syndrome
Cestoda
Cestodaria
cestode
cestodiasis
cestoid
Cestoidea
Ceylancyclostoma
CF (Chiari-Frommel syndrome cystic fibrosis)
CFP (chronic false-positive cystic fibrosis of the pancreas)
CFU-C (colony-forming unit-culture)
CFU-E (colony-forming unit-erythroid)
CFU-S (colony-forming unit-spleen)
CFWM (cancer-free white mouse)
CG (chronic glomerulonephritis)
CGD (chronic granulomatous disease)
CGL (chronic granulocytic leukemia)
CGN (chronic glomerulonephritis)
CHA (congenital hypoplastic anemia)
Chabert's disease
Chaetomium
Chagas' disease
Chagas-Cruz disease

Additional Entries

Chagasia
chagasic
chagoma
Chagres fever
chalasia
chalazodermia
chalcitis
chalcosis
    c. corneae
chalicosis
chalkitis
chamaecephaly
Championniere's disease
chancre
chancriform
chancroid
    phagedenic c.
    serpiginous c.
chancroidal
chancrous
change
    Armanni-Ebstein c.
    Crooke's c's
    Crooke-Russell c's
    harlequin color c.
chapped
Charcot-Marie atrophy
Charcot-Marie-Tooth disease
Charcot's disease
Charcot-Weiss-Barker syndrome
charley horse
Charlin's syndrome
Charlouis' disease
Charrin's disease
chaude-pisse
Chauffard's syndrome
Chauffard-Still syndrome

Chaunacanthida
Chauveau's bacillus
CHB (complete heart block)
CHD (congestive heart disease)
Cheadle's disease
Chediak-Higashi
    C-H anomaly
    C-H disease
    C H syndrome
Chediak-Steinbrinck-Higashi syndrome
cheese washer's disease
cheilitis
    actinic c.
    angular c.
    apostematous c.
    commissural c.
    exfoliativa c.
    c. glandularis
    c. glandularis apostematosa
    c. granulomatosa
    impetiginous c.
    migrating c.
    solar c.
    c. venenata
cheilocarcinoma
cheilognathopalatoschisis
cheilognathoprosoposchisis
cheilognathoschisis
cheilognathouranoschisis
cheilophagia
cheiloschisis
cheilosis
cheiragra
cheiralgia
    c. paresthetica
cheirarthritis

Additional Entries

cheirobrachialgia
cheirocinesthesia
cheiromegaly
cheiropodalgia
cheirospasm
cheminosis
chemodectoma
Cheney syndrome
Cherchevski's disease
chest
    alar c.
    barrel c.
    blast c.
    cobbler's c.
    flail c.
    flat c.
    foveated c.
    funnel c.
    keeled c.
    paralytic c.
    phthinoid c.
    pigeon c.
    pterygoid c.
    tetrahedron c.
Chester's disease
Cheyletiella
    C. blakei
    C. parasitovorax
    C. yasguri
Cheyne-Stokes asthma
CHF (congestive heart failure)
CHH (cartilage-hair hypoplasia)
Chiari-Arnold syndrome
Chiari-Budd syndrome
Chiari-Frommel syndrome
Chiari II syndrome
Chiari's syndrome
chickenpox

chickenpox *(continued)*
    c. virus
chief cell adenoma
chigger
chikungunya
    c. fever
    c. fever virus
Chilaiditi's syndrome
chilblain
childbed fever
chilitis
chill
    brass c.
    brazier's c.
    creeping c.
    nervous c.
    shaking c.
    spelter c's
    urethral c.
    zinc c.
Chilognatha
chilomastigiasis
Chilomastix
    C. mesnili
chilomastixiasis
Chilopoda
Chinese liver fluke
Chinese restaurant syndrome
chionablepsia
chip
    bone c.
    c. fracture
Chiracanthium
chirobrachialgia
chirognostic
chiromegaly
Chironomidae
Chironomus

Additional Entries

chiropodalgia
Chiroptera
chirospasm
chlamydemia
Chlamydia
    C. oculogenitalis
    C. psittaci
    C. trachomatis
Chlamydiaceae
chlamydiosis
Chlamydobacteriaceae
Chlamydobacteriales
Chlamydophrys
chlamydospore
Chlamydozoaceae
Chlamydozoon
chloasma
    c. hepaticum
chloracne
chlorhistechia
chlorhydria
chloridorrhea
chloriduria
Chlorobacterium
Chlorobiaceae
Chlorobium
chlorobrightism
chloroerythroblastoma
chloroleukemia
chlorolymphosarcoma
chloroma
chloromonad
Chloromonadida
chloromyeloma
chloropexia
chloropsia
chlorosis
Choanotaenia

Choanotaenia *(continued)*
    C. infundibulum
chocolate cyst
choke
    water c.
cholangeitis
cholangiectasis
cholangioadenoma
cholangiocarcinoma
cholangiohepatitis
cholangiohepatoma
cholangiolitic cirrhosis
cholangiolitis
cholangioma
cholangitis
    chronic nonsuppurative destructive c.
    c. lenta
    progressive nonsuppurative c.
    sclerosing c.
    suppurative c.
cholecystalgia
cholecystectasia
cholecystitis
    acute c.
    acute hemorrhagic c.
    chronic c.
    emphysematous c.
    follicular c.
    gaseous c.
    glandularis proliferans c.
cholecystolithiasis
cholecystosis
    hyperplastic c.
choledocholithiasis
cholelithiasis
cholemia

Additional Entries

cholemic nephrosis
cholepathia
cholera
    Asiatic c.
    chicken c.
    dry c.
    fowl c.
    c. gallinarium
    hog c.
    c. morbus
    pancreatic c.
    c. sicca
    summer c.
Choleraesuis
    C. salmonella
cholestasis
cholesteatoma
cholesteatomatous
cholesteatosis
cholesteremia
cholesterinemia
cholesterohistechia
cholesterolemia
cholesterolosis
cholesteroluria
cholesterosis
    extracellular c.
chondralgia
chondritis
chondroadenoma
chondroangioma
chondroblastoma
chondrocalcinosis
chondrocarcinoma
chondrodermatitis
    c. nodularis chronica
        helicis
chondrodynia

chondrodysplasia
    hereditary deforming c.
    c. punctata
chondrodystrophia
    c. calcificans congenita
chondrodystrophy
    familial c.
    hereditary deforming c.
    hyperplastic c.
    hypoplastic c.
    hypoplastic fetal c.
    c. malacia
chondroendothelioma
chondroepiphysitis
chondrofibroma
chondroid
    c. metaplasia
    c. syringoma
chondrolipoma
chondroma
    joint c.
    c. sarcomatosum
    synovial c.
    true c.
chondromalacia
    c. fetalis
    c. patellae
chondromatosis
    synovial c.
chondromatous
    c. exostosis
    c. giant cell tumor
chondrometaplasia
    synovial c.
    tenosynovial c.
chondromyoma
chondromyxoid
    c. fibroma

Additional Entries

chondromyxoma
chondromyxosarcoma
chondronecrosis
chondropathia
    c. tuberosa
chondropathology
chondropathy
chondrosarcoma
    central c.
    mesenchymal c.
chondrosarcomatosis
chondrosarcomatous
chorangioma
chorditis
    c. cantorum
    c. fibrinosa
    c. nodosa
    c. tuberosa
    c. vocalis
    c. vocalis inferior
chordoblastoma
chordocarcinoma
chordoepithelioma
chordoma
chordosarcoma
chorea
    acute c.
    Bergeron's c.
    chronic progressive
      hereditary c.
    chronic progressive
      nonhereditary c.
    c. cordis
    dancing c.
    degenerative c.
    diaphragmatic c.
    c. dimidiata
    Dubini c.

chorea *(continued)*
    electric c.
    c. festinans
    fibrillary c.
    c. gravidarum
    hemilateral c.
    Henoch's c.
    hereditary c.
    Huntington's c.
    hyoscine c.
    hysterical c.
    juvenile c.
    laryngeal c.
    limp c.
    malleatory c.
    methodic c.
    mimetic c.
    c. minor
    c. mollis
    Morvan's c.
    c. nocturnia
    c. nutans
    one-sided c.
    paralytic c.
    hemiplegic c.
    posthemiplegic c.
    prehemiplegic c.
    saltatory c.
    Schrotter's c.
    senile c.
    simple c.
    Sydenham's c.
choreoathetosis
chorioadenoma
    c. destruens
chorioamnionitis
chorioangiofibroma
chorioangioma

Additional Entries

chorioblastoma
chorioblastosis
choriocarcinoma
choriocele
chorioepithelioma
   c. malignum
chorioma
choriomeningitis
   lymphocytic c.
chorionepithelioma
chorionic carcinoma
chorioretinitis
   c. sclopetaria
   toxoplasmic c.
chorioretinopathy
choroideremia
choroiditis
   acute diffuse serous c.
   anterior c.
   areolar c.
   central c.
   diffuse c.
   disseminated c.
   Doyne's familial
     honeycombed c.
   exudative c.
   focal c.
   Forster's c.
   c. guttata senilis
   juxtapapillary c.
   macular c.
   macular exudative c.
   c. serosa
   suppurative c.
   Tay's c.
choroidocyclitis
choroidoiritis
choroidopathy

choroidoretinitis
Chotzen's syndrome
Christensen-Krabbe disease
Christian's disease
Christian-Weber disease
Christmas disease
Christ-Siemens syndrome
Christ-Siemens-Touraine
   syndrome
chromaffic
   c. paraganglioma
   c. tumor
chromaffinoma
   medullary c.
chromaffinopathy
chromatopsia
chromaturia
chromesthesia
chromhidrosis
Chromobacterium
   C. amythistinum
   C. janthinum
   C. marismortui
   C. typhiflavum
   C. violaceum
chromoblastomycosis
chromodacryorrhea
chromomycosis
chromophobe adenoma
chromorhinorrhea
chromosomal breakage
   syndrome
chromotoxic
chronic
   c. active hepatitis
   c. bronchitis
   c. granulomatous disease
   c. interstitial nephritis

Additional Entries

chronic *(continued)*
    c. lymphatic leukemia
    c. lymphocytic leukemia
    c. lymphosarcoma
      leukemia
    c. monocytic leukemia
    c. myelogenous leukemia
    c. obstructive pulmonary
      disease
    c. renal disease
    c. renal failure
    c. subdural hematoma
    c. thyroiditis
chroniosepsis
chronotaraxis
chrysiasis
Chrysomyia
    C. albiceps
    C. bezziana
    C. macellaria
Chrysops
    C. cecutiens
    C. dimidiata
    C. discalis
    C. silacea
CHS (Chediak-Higashi
  syndrome)
Churg-Strauss syndrome
Chvostek's symptom
Chvostek-Weiss sign
chylangioma
chylectasia
chylemia
chylocele
    parasitic c.
chyloderma
chylomicronemia
chylopericarditis

chylopleura
chylopneumothorax
chylorrhea
chylous
    c. ascites
    c. effusion
chyluria
CI (cerebral infarction)
Ciarrocchi's disease
CID (cytomegalic inclusion
  disease)
CIDS (cellular immunity
  deficiency syndrome)
ciliocytophthoria
cillosis
Cillobacterium
Cimex
    C. lectularius
CIN (cervical intraepithelial
  neoplasia, chronic interstitial
  nephritis)
cinesalgia
cirrhosis
    acholangic biliary c.
    acute juvenile c.
    alcoholic c.
    atrophic c.
    bacterial c.
    biliary c.
    biliary c. of children
    calculus c.
    cardiac c.
    Charcot's c.
    cholangiolitic c.
    congestive c.
    Cruveilheier-Baumgarten
      c.
    fatty c.

Additional Entries

cirrhosis *(continued)*
    Hanot's c.
    hypertrophic c.
    Indian childhood c.
    Laennec's c.
    c. of liver
    c. of lung
    malarial c.
    c. mammae
    metabolic c.
    multilobular c.
    nutritional c.
    obstructive c.
    periportal c.
    pigmentary c.
    pipestem c.
    portal c.
    posthepatic c.
    postnecrotic c.
    primary biliary c.
    pulmonary c.
    secondary biliary c.
    stasis c.
    c. of stomach
    syphilitic c.
    Todd's c.
    toxic c.
    unilobular c.
    vascular c.
cirrhotic
cirsocele
cirsomphalos
cirsophthalmia
CIS (carcinoma in situ)
Citelli's syndrome
Citrobacter
    C. amalonaticus

Citrobacter *(continued)*
    Bethesda-Ballerup group of C.
    C. diversus
    C. freundii
    C. intermedius
citrullinemia
citrullinuria
citta
cittosis
Civatte's poikiloderma
Cl. (Clostridium)
cladiosis
cladosporiosis
Cladosporium
    C. bantianum
    C. carrionii
    C. cladosporoides
    C. mansonii
    C. trichoides
    C. werneckii
Clarke-Hadfield syndrome
clasmatocytosis
clasmocytoma
Claude Bernard-Horner syndrome
Claude's hyperkinesis syndrome
claudication
    intermittent c.
    venous c.
claustrophilia
claustrophobia
clausura
clawfoot
clawhand
CLBBB (complete left bundle branch block)

Additional Entries

CLD (chronic liver disease, chronic lung disease)
clear cell
    c. c. adenocarcinoma
    c. c. adenoma
    c. c. carcinoma
    c. c. hidradenoma
    c. c. sarcoma
cleft
    c. lip
    c. nose
    c. palate
    c. tongue
Clerambault-Kandinsky syndrome
click
    ejection c.
    midsystolic c.
clitoriditis
clitorimegaly
clitoritis
clitoromegaly
CLL (chronic lymphatic leukemia, chronic lymphocytic leukemia)
cloacogenic carcinoma
clonorchiasis
Clonorchis
    C. sinensis
Clostridium
    C. bifermentans
    C. botulinum
    C. butyricum
    C. clostridiiforme
    C. difficile
    C. histolyticum
    C. histolyticum collagenase

Clostridium *(continued)*
    C. innocuum
    C. novyi
    C. perfringens
    C. ramosus
    C. septicum
    C. sordellii
    C. sphenoides
    C. tertium
    C. tetani
    C. welchii
cloudy swelling
Cloudman's melanoma S91
Clough and Richter's syndrome
Clouston's syndrome
clubbed
    c. fingers
    c. toes
clubbing
clubfoot
clubhand
    radial c.
    ulnar c.
clubroot
CMF (chondromyxoid fibroma)
CMGN (chronic membranous glomerulonephritis)
CMID (cytomegalic inclusion disease)
CML (chronic myelogenous leukemia)
CMM (cutaneous malignant melanoma)
CMN (cystic medial necrosis)
CMN-AA (cystic medial necrosis of the ascending aorta)
CMoL (chronic monocytic (monoblastic) leukemia)

Additional Entries

CMP (cardiomyopathy)
CNHD (congenital nonspherocytic hemolytic disease)
CO (corneal opacity)
coagulative necrosis
coal worker's pneumoconiosis
coarctation
    c. of aorta
        postductal c. of aorta
        preductal c. of aorta
        reversed c.
Coat's disease
cobaltosis
cobbler's chest
cobraism
cocarcinogen
cocarcinogenesis
cocci
Coccidia
coccidioidal
    c. granuloma
Coccidioides
    C. immitis
coccidioidoma
coccidioidomycosis
    primary extrapulmonary c.
coccidiosis
Coccidium
    C. hominis
coccidium
Coccobacillus
coccobacillus
coccobacteria
coccoid
coccus
coccyalgia
coccygodynia

coccyodynia
Cockayne's syndrome
cockscomb polyp
Codman's tumor
Coffin-Lowry syndrome
Coffin-Siris syndrome
Cogan's syndrome
cogwheel respiration
coin lesion
COLD (chronic obstructive lung disease)
cold
    c. agglutinin syndrome
    c. hemoglobinuria
    c. injury
    c. intoleracne
    c. lesion
coldsore
Cole's sign
colibacillemia
colibacillosis
    C. gravidarum
colibacilluria
colibacillus
colic
    appendicular c.
    biliary c.
    bilious c.
    copper c.
    Devonshire c.
    endemic c.
    flatulent c.
    gallstone c.
    infantile c.
    intestinal c.
    lead c.
    menstrual c.
    nephric c.

Additional Entries

colic *(continued)*
    ovarian c.
    painter's c.
    pancreatic c.
    Poitu c.
    renal c.
    saturnine c.
    stercoral c.
    tubal c.
    ureteral c.
    uterine c.
    vermicular c.
    verminous c.
    wind c.
    worm c.
    zinc c.
colica
    c. pictonum
    c. scortorum
colicky
colicoplegia
colicystitis
colicystopyelitis
colinephritis
colitis
    acute ulcerative c.
    amebic c.
    antibiotic-associated c.
    balantidial c.
    chronic ulcerative c.
    c. cystica profunda
    c. cystica superficia
    granulomatous c.
    c. gravis
    ischemic c.
    mucous c.
    c. polyposa
    pseudomembranous c.

colitis *(continued)*
    radiation c.
    regional c.
    segmental c.
    spastic c.
    transmural c.
    c. ulcerative
    uremic c.
colitoxemia
colitoxicosis
colitoxin
coliuria
collagen disease
Collet-Sicard syndrome
Collet's syndrome
colloid
    c. adenocarcinoma
    c. adenoma
    c. carcinoma
    c. cyst
    c. degeneration
    c. goiter
colloidoclasia
coloboma
    atypical c.
    bridge c.
    c. of choroid
    c. of ciliary body
    complete c.
    Fuchs's c.
    c. of fundus
    c. lobuli
    c. of optic disk
    c. of optic nerve
    c. at optic nerve entrance
    c. palpebrale
    peripapillary c.
    c. of retinae

Additional Entries

coloboma *(continued)*
    retinochoroidal c.
    typical c.
    c. of vitreous
colonalgia
colonitis
colonopathy
colonorrhagia
colopathy
coloptosis
Colorado
    C. tick fever
    C. tick fever virus
color blindness
colorectitis
colpagia
colpatresia
colpectasia
colpitis
colpocele
colpocystitis
colpocystocele
colpodynia
colpohyperplasia
    c. cystica
    c. emphysematosa
colpoperineorrhaphy
colpoptosis
colporrhagia
colporrhexis
colpolspasm
colpostenosis
colpoxerosis
Columbia-SK virus
coma
    agrypnodal c.
    alcoholic c.
    alpha c.

coma *(continued)*
    apoplectic c.
    c. de passe
    diabetic c.
    hepatic c.
    hyperosmolar nonketotic c.
    irreversible c.
    Kussmaul's c.
    metabolic c.
    c. somnolentium
    uremic c.
    c. vigil
Comamonas terrigena
comatose
comedocarcinoma
comedomastitis
commotio
    c. cerebri
    c. retinae
    c. spinalis
Comolli's sign
compaction
compensation neurosis
compensatory
    c. emphysema
    c. hypertrophy
complete
    c. anomalous venous drainage
    c. heart block
    c. right bundle branch block
complex
    c. adrenal endocrine disorder
    AIDS-related c. (ARC)

Additional Entries

complex *(continued)*
    amyotrophic lateral
        sclerosis-parkinsonism-
        dementia c.
    anomalous c.
    Eisenmenger c.
    c. gonadal endocrine
        disorder
    c. odontoma
    c. pituitary endocrine
        disorder
    primary c.
    primary tuberculous c.
    sicca c.
    symptom c.
    c. thyroid endocrine
        disorder
composite tumor
compound
    c. leukemia
    c. nevus
    c. odontoma
    c. tumor
compression
    c. of the brain
    digital c.
    spinal c.
compulsion
    repetition c.
Concato's disease
conchiolinosteomyelitis
conchitis
concretio
    c. cordis
    c. pericardii
concretion
    alvine c.
    calculous c.

concretion *(continued)*
    preputial c.
    prostatic c's
    tophic c.
concussion
    abdominal c.
    air c.
    c. of the brain
    c. of the labyrinth
    pulmonary c.
    c. of the retina
    c. of the spinal cord
conduction
    c. deafness
    c. defect
    delayed c.
    ephaptic c.
condylarthrosis
condyloma
    c. acuminatum
    giant c. of Buschke-
        Lowenstein
    c. latum
    pointed c.
condylomata
condylomatoid
condylomatosis
condylomatous
confluent
    c. bronchopneumonia
    c. inflammation
    c. pneumonia
congenital
    c. adrenal hyperplasia
    c. nonspherocytic
        hemolytic disease
    c. thymic dysplasia
congestion

Additional Entries

congestion *(continued)*
    active c.
    functional c.
    hypostatic c.
    neuroparalytic c.
    neurotonic c.
    passive c.
    physiologic c.
    pulmonary c.
    venous c.
congestive
    c. cirrhosis
    c. edema
    c. heart failure
coniofibrosis
coniolymphstasis
coniosis
Coniosporium
coniosporosis
coniotoxicosis
conjunctivitis
    actinic c.
    acute catarrhal c.
    acute contagious c.
    acute hemorrhagic c.
    adult gonococcal c.
    allergic c.
    angular c.
    arc-flash c.
    atopic c.
    atropine c.
    blennorrheal c.
    calcareous c.
    catarrhal c.
    chemical c.
    chronic catarrhal c.
    croupous c.
    diphtheritic c.

conjunctivitis *(continued)*
    diplobacillary c.
    eczematous c.
    Egyptian c.
    epidemic c.
    follicular c.
    gonococcal c.
    granular c.
    inclusion c.
    infantile purulent c.
    Koch-Weeks c.
    larval c.
    lithiasis c.
    medicamentosis c.
    membranous c.
    meningococcus c.
    molluscum c.
    Morax-Axenfeld c.
    necrotic infectious c.
    c. neonatorum
    c. nodosa
    Parinaud's c.
    Pascheff's c.
    c. petrificans
    phlyctenular c.
    prairie c.
    pseudomembranous c.
    purulent c.
    scrofular c.
    shipyard c.
    simple c.
    simple acute c.
    spring catarrhal c.
    swimming pool c.
    trachomatous c.
    tularemic c.
    uratic c.
    vaccinial c.

Additional Entries

conjunctivitis *(continued)*
    vernal c.
    welder's c.
    Widmark's c.
conjunctivoma
Conn's syndrome
conophthalmus
Conor and Bruch's disease
Conradi's disease
constipation
constitutional
    c. dwarf
    c. hyperbilirubinemia
    c. thrombopathy
constriction
constrictive
consumption
    c. coagulopathy
    galloping c.
    luxus c.
contact dermatitis
contracted kidney
contracture
    congenital c.
    Dupuytren's c.
    ischemic c.
    organic c.
    postpoliomyelitic c.
    veratrin c.
    Volkmann's c.
contrafissure
contralateral
    c. axillary metastasis
contrecoup
contusion
    contrecoup c.
conversion hysteria
convulsion

convulsion *(continued)*
    central c.
    clonic c.
    coordinate c.
    crowing c.
    epileptiform c.
    essential c.
    febrile c.
    hysterical c.
    local c.
    mimetic c.
    puerperal c.
    salaam c.
    spontaneous c.
    tetanic c.
    tonic c.
    uremic c.
convulsive
Cooley's anemia
Cooper's
    C. disease
    C. irritable breast
Coopernail's sign
COPD (chronic obstructive pulmonary disease)
copiopia
copodyskinesia
copracrasia
copremesis
Coprococcus
coprolagnia
coprolith
Copromastix
    C. prowazeki
Copromonas
    C. subtilis
coprophagia
coproporphyria

Additional Entries

coproporphyrinuria
coprostasis
cor
    c. adiposum
    c. arteriosum
    c. biloculare
    c. bovinum
    c. pendulum
    c. pseudotriloculare biatriatum
    c. pulmonale
    c. triatriatum
    c. triloculare biatriatum
    c. triloculare biventriculare
    c. villosum
coracoiditis
Corbus' disease
Cordylobia
    C. anthropophaga
corectasis
corectopia
corestenoma
    c. congenitum
Cori's disease
cornea
    conical c.
    c. farinata
    flat c.
    c. globosa
    c. guttata
    c. opaca
    c. plana
    c. verticillata
corneitis
Cornelia de Lange's syndrome
corneoiritis
coronaritis
coronary
    c. artery disease
    c. atherosclerotic heart disease
    c. heart disease
    c. insufficiency
    c. thrombosis
coronavirus
corpus
    c. hemorrhagicum
    c. hemorrhagicum cyst
Corrigan's disease
cortical
    c. defect
    c. necrosis
    c. stromal hyperplasia
corticopleuritis
Corvisart's disease
corybantism
Corynebacterium
    C. acnes
    C. belfantii
    C. diphtheriae
    C. enzymicum
    C. equi
    C. hemolyticum
    C. hoagii
    C. hofmannii
    C. infantisepticum
    C. minutissimum
    C. mycetoides
    C. necrophorum
    C. parvulum
    C. pseudodiphtheriticum
    C. pseudotuberculosis-ovis
    C. renale
    C. tenuis

Additional Entries

Corynebacterium *(continued)*
    C. ulcerans
    C. vaginale
    C. xerosis
corynebacterium
    group JK c.
    group 3 c.
coryza
    allergic c.
    c. foetida
    infectious avian c.
    c. oedematosa
coryzavirus
Costen's syndrome
Cotard's syndrome
cottonpox
Cottunius' disease
Cotugno's disease
cough
    aneurysmal c.
    Balme's c.
    barking c.
    compression c.
    dry c.
    ear c.
    extrapulmonary c.
    hacking c.
    mechanical c.
    Morton's c.
    privet c.
    productive c.
    reflex c.
    stomach c.
    Sydenham's c.
    tea taster's c.
    trigeminal c.
    wet c.
    whooping c.

cough *(continued)*
    winter c.
Councilmania
    C. dissimilis
    C. lafleuri
coup
    c. de fouet
    c. de sabre
    c. de sang
    c. de soleil
    c. sur coup
Courvoisier-Terrier syndrome
Couvelaire uterus
Cowden disease
Cowdria
    C. ruminantium
cowperitis
cowpox virus
coxalgia
coxarthria
coxarthritis
coxarthrocace
coxarthropathy
coxarthrosis
Coxiella
    C. burnetii
coxitis
    c. fugax
    senile c.
coxodynia
coxotuberculosis
coxsackievirus
    c. A
    c. B
CP (cerebral palsy)
CPN (chronic pyelonephritis)
crackle
    pleural c's

Additional Entries

_____
_____
_____
_____
_____

cramp
    accessory c.
    heat c.
    recumbency c.'s
    stoker's c.
    writer's c.
Crandall's syndrome
cranial arteritis
craniofenestria
craniolacunia
craniomalacia
craniomeningocele
craniopagus
    c. occipitalis
    c. parasiticus
    c. parietalis
craniopathy
    metabolic c.
craniopharyngioma
craniorachischisis
cranioschisis
craniosclerosis
craniostenosis
craniostosis
craniosynostosis
craniotabes
craniotrypesis
cranitis
cranium
    c. bifidum
    c. bifidum occultum
crapulent
crapulous
craw-craw
CRBBB (complete right bundle branch block)
CRD (chronic renal disease)
creatinemia

creatinuria
creatorrhea
crepitation
crepitus
    articular c.
    bony c.
    false c.
    c. indux
    joint c.
    c. redux
    silken c.
crescentic glomerulopathy
cretinism
    athyreotic c.
    goitrous c.
    spontaneous c.
    sporadic goitrous c.
    sporadic nongoitrous c.
cretinistic
cretinoid
cretinous
Creutzfeldt-Jakob disease
Crichton-Browne's sign
cricoidynia
CRF (chronic renal failure)
cribiform carcinoma
cri du chat syndrome
Crigler-Najjar syndrome
Crimean hemorrhagic fever virus
crinophagy
crisis
    addisonian c.
    adrenal c.
    anaphylactoid c.
    aplastic c.
    blast c.
    bronchial c.

Additional Entries

crisis *(continued)*
    cardiac c.
    catathymic c.
    celiac c.
    cholinergic c.
    clitoris c.
    deglobulinization c.
    Dietl's c.
    false c.
    febrile c.
    gastric c.
    genital c. of newborn
    glaucomatocyclitic c.
    hepatic c.
    identity c.
    intestinal c.
    laryngeal c.
    myasthenic c.
    nefast c.
    nephralgic c.
    nitritoid c.
    ocular c.
    oculogyric c.
    parkinsonian c.
    Pel's c.
    pharyngeal c.
    rectal c.
    renal c.
    salt-depletion c.
    salt-losing c.
    tabetic c.
    thoracic c.
    thyroid c.
    vesical c.
    visceral c.
crispation
Crocq's disease
Crohn's disease
Cronkhite-Canada synrome
Cronkhite's syndrome
Crooke's
    C. changes
    C. hyaline degeneration
cross-eye
croup
    catarrhal c.
    diphtheritic c.
    false c.
    membranous c.
    pseudomembranous c.
    spasmodic c.
croupous
Crouzon's
    C. craniofacial dysostosis disease
crowding effect
CRS (Chinese restaurant syndrome)
CRST (calcinosis cutis, Raynaud's phenomenom, sclerodactyly and telangiectasia)
crush
    c. injury
    c. kidney
    c. syndrome
Cruveilhier-Baumgarten syndrome
Cruveilhier's atrophy disease
Cruz-Chagas disease
Cruz's trypanosomiasis
cry
    arthritic c.
    cepahlic c.
    epileptic c.
    hydrocephalic c.

Additional Entries

cry *(continued)*
    joint c.
    night c.
cryalgesia
cryanesthesia
crymodynia
cryofibrinogenemia
cryoglobulinemia
cryohydrocytosis
cryopathic hemolytic syndrome
cryptitis
Cryptococcaceae
cryptococcal meningitis
cryptococci
cryptococcosis
Cryptococcus
    C. albidus/albidus
    C. albidus/diffluens
    C. capsulatus
    C. epidermidis
    C. gilchristi
    C. histolyticus
    C. hominis
    C. laurentii
    C. luteolus
    C. meningitidis
    C. neoformans
    C. terreus
cryptoglioma
cryptoleukemia
cryptolith
cryptomenorrhea
cryptomerorachischisis
cryptomnesia
cryptophthalmos
cryptopodia
cryptorchidism
cryptorchism

cryptosporiodiosis
Cryptostroma
    C. corticale
cryptostromosis
cryptotia
cryptoxanthin
cryptozygous
crystal
    asthma c's
    blood c's
    Charcot-Leyden c's
    c. deposition disease
    leukocytic c's
crystalluria
C & S (culture and sensitivity)
CSH (chronic subdural
    hematoma, cortical stromal
    hyperplasia)
Csillag's disease
CSR (Cheyne-Stokes
    respiration)
CT (coronary thrombosis)
CTD (congenital thymic
    dysplasia)
CUC (chronic ulcerative colitis)
Cunninghamella
    C. bertholletiae
    C. elegans
cupremia
Curling's ulcer
Curschmann's disease
Curtius' syndrome
Curvularia
    C. geniculata
Cushing's
    basophilism
    disease
    syndrome

Additional Entries

Cushing's *(continued)*
    ulcer
cushingoid
cutaneous malformation
CVA (cardiovascular accident, cerebrovascular accident)
CVD (cardiovascular disease)
CVH (combined ventricular hypertrophy, common variable hypogammaglobulinemia)
C virus (Coxsackie virus)
CVOD (cerebrovascular obstructive disease)
CVRD (cardiovascular renal disease)
CWDF (cell wall-deficient bacterial forms)
CWP (coal worker's pneumoconiosis)
Cyanobacteria
cyanopia
cyanosis
cyclitis
    heterochromic c.
    plastic c.
    pure c.
    purulent c.
    serous c.
cyclochoroiditis
cyclodamia
cyclokeratosis
cyclomastopathy
cyclophoria
    accommodative c.
    minus c.
    plus c.
cyclopia
cycloplegia
cycloplegic
cyclops
    c. hypognathus
cyclosis
cyclothymia
cyclotropia
cylindrathrosis
cylindrical bronchiectasis
cylindroma
    dermal eccrine c.
cylindruria
cyllosis
cyllosoma
cynanche
    c. maligna
    c. tonsillaris
Cyriax's syndrome
cyst
    adventitious c.
    allantoic c.
    alveolar c's
    alveolar hydatid c.
    amnionic c.
    aneurysmal bone c.
    angioblastic c.
    apical c.
    apoplectic c.
    arachnoid c.
    atheromatous c.
    Baker's c.
    Bartholin's c.
    Blessig's c.
    blue dome c.
    Boyer's c.
    branchial c.
    branchial cleft c.
    bronchial c.

Additional Entries

cyst *(continued)*
    bronchogenic c.
    bronchiopulmonary c.
    chocolate c.
    choledochal c.
    choledochus c.
    chyle c.
    colloid c.
    compound c.
    congenital c.
    corpus hemorrhagicum c.
    corpus luteum c.
    craniobuccal c.
    craniopharyngeal c.
    daughter c.
    dental follicular c.
    dentigerous c.
    dermoid c.
    dilatation c.
    distention c.
    echinococcus c.
    embryonal duct c.
    endometrial c.
    endothelial c.
    enteric c.
    ependymal c.
    epidermal c.
    epidermal inclusion c.
    epidermoid c.
    epidermoid inclusion c.
    epididymal c.
    epithelial c.
    epithelial inclusion c.
    eruption c.
    extravasation c.
    exudation c.
    false c.
    fissural c.

cyst *(continued)*
    follicle c.
    follicular c.
    ganglion c.
    Gartner's duct c.
    gas c.
    germinal epithelial
        inclusion c.
    germinal inclusion c.
    gingival c.
    globulomaxillary c.
    granddaughter c.
    hemorrhagic c.
    hydatid c.
    implantation c.
    incisive canal c.
    inclusion c.
    inflammatory c.
    intraepithelial c.
    keratinous c.
    intraluminal c.
    intrapituitary c.
    involution c.
    Iwanoff's c.
    keratinizing c.
    Kobelt's c.
    lacteal c.
    lateral periodontal c.
    leptomeningeal c
    luteal c.
    luteinized follicular c.
    median anterior maxillary
        c.
    median mandibular c.
    median palatal c.
    meibomian c.
    mesenteric c.
    mesonephric c.

Additional Entries

cyst *(continued)*
- mesothelial c.
- milk c.
- milum c.
- Morgagni's c.
- mucinous c.
- mucous c.
- multilocular c.
- myxoid c.
- nabothian c.
- nasoalveolar c.
- nasopalatine duct c.
- necrotic c.
- neural c.
- neurenteric c.
- nevoid c.
- odontogenic c.
- omental c.
- oophoritic c.
- osseous hydatid c's
- pancreatic c.
- paranephric c.
- parapyelitic c's
- paraphyseal c.
- parasitic c.
- parathyroid c.
- pearl c.
- periapical c.
- pericardial c.
- perineural c.
- periodontal c.
- pilar c.
- pilonidal c.
- placental c.
- porencephalic c.
- preauricular c.
- primordial c.
- pseudomucinous c.

cyst *(continued)*
- pyelogenic renal c.
- radicular c.
- ranular c.
- Rathke's c.
- renal c.
- retention c.
- Sampson's c.
- sanguineous c.
- sebaceous c.
- serous c.
- simple c.
- soapsuds c's
- solitary c.
- springwater c.
- sterile c.
- subchondral c.
- sublingual c.
- subsynovial c.
- suprasellar c.
- synovial c.
- Tarlov c.
- tarry c.
- tarsal c.
- tension c.
- thecal c.
- theca-lutein c.
- tissue c.
- thymic c's
- thyroglossal duct c.
- Tornwaldt's c.
- trichilemmal c.
- true c.
- tubular c.
- umbilical c.
- unicameral c.
- unicameral bone c.
- unilocular c.

Additional Entries

cyst *(continued)*
    urinary c.
    vitellointestinal c.
    wolffian c.
cystadenocarcinoma
    mucinous c.
    papillary c.
    papillary serous c.
    pseudomucinous c.
    serous c.
cystadenofibroma
cystadenoma
    c. adamantinum
    c. lymphomatosum
    mucinous c.
    oncocytic papillary c.
    papillary c.
    papillary c, lymphomatosum
    papillary serous c.
    c. partim simplex
    pseudomucinous c.
    serous c.
cystalgia
cystathioninuria
cystatrophia
cystauchenitis
cystectasia
cystelcosis
cystencephalus
cysterethism
cysthypersarcosis
cystic
    c. acute inflammation
    c. atrophy
    c. chronic cervicitis
    c. chronic inflammation
    c. corpus hemorrhagicum

cystic *(continued)*
    c. degeneration
    c. dermoid teratoma
    c. disease
    c. endometrial hyperplasia
    c. fibrosis
    c. granulomatous inflammation
    c. hygroma
    c. hyperplasia
    c. inflammation
    c. mastitis
    c. mastopathy
    c. medial necrosis
    c. medionecrosis
cysticercosis
Cysticerus
    C. acanthrotrias
    C. bovis
    C. cellulosae
    C. fasciolaris
    C. ovis
    C. tenuicollis
cysticercus
cystigerous
cystinemia
cystinosis
cystinuria
cystirrhagia
cystirrhea
cystistaxis
cystitis
    acute hemorrhagic c.
    allergic c.
    bacterial c.
    catarrhal c., acute
    c. colli
    croupous c.

Additional Entries

cystitis *(continued)*
    c. cystica
    diphtheritic c.
    c. emphysematosa
    eosinophilic c.
    exfoliative c.
    c. follicularis
    c. glandularis
    hemorrhagic c.
    Hunner's c.
    incrusted c.
    interstitial c., chronic
    mechanical c.
    panmural c.
    c. papillomatosa
    c. pneumatoides
    c. senilis feminarum
    submucous c.
    ulcerative c.
cystoadenoma
Cystobacter
cystocarcinoma
cystocele
cystodynia
cystoenterocele
cystoepiplocele
cestoepithelioma
cystofibroma
cystolith
cystolithiasis
cystoma
    serous c.
cystomatitis
cystomatous
cystomyoma
cystomyxoadenoma
cystomyxoma
cystonephrosis

cystoneuralgia
cystoparalysis
cystophthisis
cystoplegia
cystoptosis
cystopyelitis
cystopyelonephritis
cystorrhagia
cystorrhea
cystosarcoma
    c. phyllodes
    c. phylloides
cystoschiosis
cystosclerosis
cystospasm
cystospermitis
cystostaxis
cystoureteritis
cystoureteropyelitis
cystoureteropyelonephritis
cystourethritis
cystourethrocele
Cytauxzoon
    C. felis
cytauxzoonosis
cytochalasin
    c. B
cytoclasis
cytoclastic
cytokalipenia
cytoma
cytomegalic
    c. inclusion disease
    c. inclusion disease virus
cytomegalovirus
cytomegaly
cyptopathic
cytopathogenesis

Additional Entries

cytopathogenic
cytopathology
cytopenia
cytostasis
cytotoxic

c. necrosis
cytotoxicity
Cytotoxan
Czerny's disease

Additional Entries

Additional Entries

D

DA (degenerative arthritis)
DaCosta's syndrome
dacryoadenitis
dacryoblennorrhea
dacryocyst
dacryocystitis
DAH (disordered action of the heart)
damage
    irradiation d.
    radiation d.
dandruff
dandy fever
Dandy-Walker syndrome
Darier's disease
Darling's disease
deafness
    conduction d.
    high frequency d.
    mixed-type d.
    nerve d.
    tone d.
death
    brain d.
    cell d.
    crib d.
    fetal d.
    d. fever
    functional d.
    natural d.
Debaryomyces
    D. hansenii
    D. hominis
    D. neoformans

debrancher deficiency limit dextrinosis
decidual metaplasia
decompensation
    cardiac d.
    d. injury
    d. sickness
decompression sickness
decrementing response
decubitus ulcer
defect
    acquired d.
    atrial septal d.
    congenital d.
    ectodermal d.
    endocardial cushion d's
    fibrous cortical d.
    neural tube d.
    septal d.
    surgical d.
    ventricular septal d.
defibrination syndrome
deficiency
    d. disease
    vitamin d.
deformity
    acquired d.
    congenital d.
    Klippel-Feil d.
    lobster claw d.
    pigeon breast d.
    valgus d.
    varus d.
degenerated
    d. intervertebral disc

Additional Entries

degenerated *(continued)*
    d. intervertebral
        fibrocartilage
    d. meniscus
degenerating
    d. myelin demonstration
degeneration
    albuminous d.
    amyloid d.
    ascending d.
    axonal d.
    ballooning d.
    basophilic d.
    calcareous d.
    cellular d.
    cloudy swelling d.
    collagen d.
    colloid d.
    Crooke's hyaline d.
    cystic d.
    cystoid d.
    cytologic d.
    descending d.
    fatty d.
    feathery d.
    fibrinoid d.
    fibrinous d.
    floccular d.
    granular d.
    hepatolenticular d.
    hyaline d.
    hydatid d.
    hydropic d.
    lipid d.
    lipoid d.
    liquefactive d.
    medial d.
    mucinous d.

degeneration *(continued)*
    mucoid d.
    myelin d.
    myxoid d.
    myxomatous d.
    parenchymatous d.
    pigmentary d.
    pseudomucinous d.
    secondary d.
    subacute combined d.
    trans-synaptic d.
    wallerian d.
    waxy d.
    Zenker's d.
degenerative
    d. arthritis
    d. change
    d. index
dehiscence
dehydration
Dejerine-Sottas disease
de Lange's syndrome
delayed
    d. adrenarche
    d. climacteric
    d. hypersensitivity
        reaction
    d. menopause
    d. puberty
delirium
dementia
    presenile d.
    senile d.
demyelinating disease
demyelination
demyelinization
dengue
    hemorrhagic d.

Additional Entries

dengue *(continued)*
    d. virus, types 1, 2, 3, 4
dental
    d. calculus
    d. caries
    d. follicular cyst
    d. granuloma
    d. plaque
dentigerous
    d. cyst
    d. mixed tumor
dentin dysplasia
dentinogenesis imperfecta
dentinoma
    fibroameloblastic d.
depigmentation
deplasmolysis
deposition
    malarial pigment d.
    xanthomatous d.
depressed
    d. fracture
    d.-type manic-depressive psychosis
depression
    psychoneurotic d.
    reactive d.
deQuervain's
    d. disease
    d. thyroiditis
Dercum's disease
Dermacentor
    D. andersoni
    D. occidentalis
    D. reticulatus
    D. variabilis
Dermacentroxenus
    D. sibericus

dermal
    d. eccrine cylindroma
    d. epidermal nevus
    d. nevus
Dermanyssus
    D. gallinae
dermatitis
    actinic d.
    allergic d.
    atopic d.
    d. atrophicans
    d. atrophicans diffusa
    d. atrophicans maculosa
    chronica atrophicans idiopathica d.
    contact d.
    eczematoid d.
    d. escharotica
    exfoliative d.
    factitious d.
    d. gangrenosa infantum
    d. herpetiformis
    lichenoid d.
    d. medicamentosa
    photo contact d.
    phototoxic contact d.
    pigmented purpuric lichenoid d.
    psoriasiform d.
    radiation d.
    d. repens
    seborrheic d.
    stasis d.
    toxic d.
    d. venenata
Dermatobia
    D. hominis
dermatofibroma

Additional Entries

dermatofibrosarcoma
    d. protuberans
dermatofibrosis
    d. lenticularis disseminata
dermatomycosis
dermatomyositis
dermatopathic
    d. lymphadenitis
    d. lymphadenopathy
dermatophilosis
Dermatophilus
    D. congolensis
    D. penetrans
dermatophytosis
dermatosis
    progressive pigmentary d.
dermoid cyst
dermopathy
deuteranomaly
deuteranopia
deuterohemophilia
Deuteromycetes
developmental jaw cyst
Devic's disease
dextrocardia
    isolated d.
dextrosuria
DFU (dead fetus in utero)
DHL (diffuse histocytic lymphoma)
dhobie itch
DI (diabetes insipidus)
diabetes
    bronzed d.
    d. insipidus
    juvenile-onset d.
    d. mellitus
diabetic

diabetic *(continued)*
    d. angiopathy
    d. coma
    d. dermopathy
    d. glomerulosclerosis
    hyperosmolar d. coma
    d. ketoacidosis
    d. lipemia
    d. myelopathy
    d. retinopathy
diakinesis
Diamond-Blackfan anemia
diaphragmatic hernia
diarrhea
diastolic
    d. hypertension
    d. murmur
diathesis
    hemorrhagic d.
Dicrocoelium
    D. dendriticum
diencephalic syndrome
Dientamoeba
    D. fragilis
diffuse
    d. acute inflammation
    d. acute peritonitis
    d. amyloidosis
    d. bronchopneumonia
    d. chronic inflammation
    d. enlargement
    d. esophageal spasm
    d. fibrosis
    d. hyperplasia
    d. hypertrophy
    d. illumination
    d. interstitial fibrosis
    d. lymphatic tissue

Additional Entries

diffuse *(continued)*
    d. meningiomatosis
    d. necrosis
    d. pneumonia
    d. pyelonephritis
    d. septal cirrhosis
    d. ulceration
DiGeorge's syndrome
digestive disorder
Di Guglielmo's syndrome
diktyoma
Dimastigamoeba
Dinobdella
    D. ferox
Dioctophyma
    D. renale
DIP (desquamative interstitial pneumonia, desquamative interstitial pneumonitis)
Dipetalonema
    D. perstans
    D. streptocerca
dipetalonemiasis
diphasic
    d. meningoencephalitis virus
    d. milk fever virus
diphtheria
diphtheroid
    aerobic d.
    anaerobic d.
    d. bacilli
diphyllobothriasis
Diphyllobothrium
    D. latum
diplegia
diplobacillus
diplobacterium

Diplococcus
    D. constellatus
    D. magnus
    D. morbillorum
    D. mucosus
    D. paleopneumoniae
    D. plagarumbelli
    D. pneumoniae
diplococcus
    d. of Morax-Axenfeld
    d. of Neisser
    Weichselbaum's d.
Diplogaster
Diplogonoporus
    D. brauni
    D. grandis
diplonema
diplopia
dipygus
    d. parasiticus
Dipylidium
    D. caninum
direct hernia
Dirofilaria
    D. conjunctivae
    D. immitis
    D. repens
    D. tenuis
dirofilariasis
discoid lupus erythematosus
disorder
    functional d.
    intestinal flow d.
    ion d.
    peristalsis d.
    ureteral peristalsis d.
disproportion
    cephalopelvic d.

Additional Entries

dissecting aneurysm
disseminated
    d. acute lupus
      erythematosus
    d. inflammation
    d. intravascular
      coagulation
    d. lupus erythematosus
    d. sclerosis
distal
    d. latency
    d. myopathy
    d.-type progressive
      muscular dystrophy
Distoma
distomiasis
disuse atrophy
diverticulitis
    hemorrhagic d.
    obstructive d.
    perforated d.
diverticulosis
diverticulum
    colonic d.
    epiphrenic d.
    false d.
    intestinal d.
    Meckel's d.
    pharyngoesophageal d.
    pressure d.
    pulsion d.
    traction d.
    Zenker's d.
dizziness
DJD (degenerative joint disease)
DK (diseased kidney)
DLE (discoid lupus
  erythematosus)

DM (diabetes mellitus, diastolic
  murmur)
DMD (Duchenne's muscular
  dystrophy)
docimasia
    auricular d.
    hepatic d.
    pulmonary d.
DOE (dyspnea on exercise,
  dyspnea on exertion)
Dohle-Heller aortitis
Dolichos
    D. biflorus
Donohue's syndrome
Donovania
    D. granulomatis
DPD (diffuse pulmonary
  disease)
DPDL (diffuse, poorly
  differentiated lymphoma)
DR (diabetic retinopathy)
dracontiasis
dracunculiasis
dracunculosis
Dracunculus
    D. medinesis
dragon worm infection
Drechslera hawaiiensis
Drepanidotaenia
    D. lanceolata
drepanocytemia
drepanocytic
drepanocytosis
Drepanospira
Drosophila
dry
    d. catarrh
    d. gangrene

Additional Entries

DS (Down's syndrome)
DSAP (disseminated superficial actinic porokeratosis)
Dubin-Johnson syndrome
Duchenne's
    disease
    -type muscular dystrophy
Ducrey's bacillus
Dumdum fever
dumping syndrome
duodenal ulcer
duovirus
Dupuytren's
    contracture
    fibromatosis
Duttonella
dwarf
    achondroplastic d.
    constitutional d.
    pituitary d.
    primordial d.
    d. tapeworm
dwarfism
    pituitary d.
dysarthria
dysaudia
dysautonomia
    familial d.
dysbarism
dysbasia
dysbetalipoproteinemia
    familial d.
dysbolism
dyschezia
dyschondroplasia
dyscrasia
    blood d.
    lymphatic d.

dysdiadochokinesia
dysdiemorrhysis
dysentery
    amebic d.
    bacillary d.
    balantidial d.
    bilharzial d.
    catarrhal d.
    ciliary d.
    ciliate d.
    epidemic d.
    flagellate d.
    Flexner's d.
    fulminant d.
    giardiasis d.
    malarial d.
    protozoal d.
    scorbutic d.
    Sonne d.
    spirillar d.
    sporadic d.
    viral d.
dyserythropoiesis
dyserythropoietic
    d. congenital anemia
dysfibrinogenemia
dysfunction
    constitutional hepatic d.
    uterine d.
    vasomotor d.
dysfunctional bleeding
dysgammaglobulinemia
dysgenesis
    familial gonadal d.
dysgenetic
dysgerminoma
dysglobulinemia
dysgonic

Additional Entries

dyshesion
dyshidrosis
dyshormonogenesis
dyskaryosis
dyskeratosis
    d. congenita
    hereditary benign
        intraepithelial d.
dyskinesia
    tardive d.
dyslexia
dyslipoproteinemia
dysmenorrhea
dysmentation
dysmorphism
dysmyelopoietic syndrome
dysostosis
    cleidocranialis d.
    Crouzon's craniofacial d.
dyspareunia
dyspepsia
dysphagia
    sideropenic d.
dysphasia
dysphonia
dysphoria
dysplasia
    acquired d.
    chondroectodermal d.
    dentin d.
    fibrous d.
    fibrous familial d.
    fibrous monostotic d.
    fibrous polyostotic d.
    hereditary d., ectodermal
    mammary d.

dysplasia *(continued)*
    polyostotic fibrous d.
    precancerous d.
    thymic d.
    vesical d.
    Zenker's d.
dyspnea
    cardiac d.
    exertional d.
    paroxysmal d.
    paroxysmal nocturnal d.
dyspneic
dyspoiesis
dysprosium
dysproteinemia
dysprothrombinemia
dysrhythmia
dyssynergia
    progressive cerebellar d.
dystaxia
dystocia
dystonia
dystonic
dystrophic
dystrophy
    adiposogenital d.
    Becker's d.
    distal muscular d.
    Duchenne-type muscular d.
    d.-dystocia syndrome
    facioscapulohumeral muscular d.
    Landouzy-Dejerine progressive muscular d.

Additional Entries

E

E. (Entamoeba, Escherichia)
EAC (Ehrlich ascites carcinoma)
EAE (experimental allergic encephalomyelitis)
Eagle syndrome
EAHF (Eczema, asthma, hay fever)
Eales's disease
EAN (experimental allergic neuritis)
eastern
    e. equine encephalitis
    e. equine encephalomyelitis virus
Eaton-Lambert syndrome
EB (epidermolysis bullosa, Epstein-Barr)
Eberthella
    E. typhi
EBL (estimated blood loss)
Ebola virus
Ebstein's
    anomaly
    disease
    malformation
EBV (Epstein-Barr virus)
EC (Escherichia coli)
ECBO virus (enteric cytopathogenic bovine orphan virus)
ecchondroma
ecchordosis physalifora
ecchymosis
eccrine
    e. poroma

eccrine *(continued)*
    e. spiradenoma
ECDO virus (enteric cytopathogenic dog orphan virus)
ECF-A (eosinophil chemotactic factor of anaphylaxis)
Echinochasmus
    E. perfoliatus
echinococciasis
echinococcosis
Echinococcus
    E. granulosus
    E. multiocularis
echinocytosis
Echinorhynchus
echinosis
Echinostoma
    E. cinetorchis
    E. ilocanum
    E. lindoensis
    E. malayanum
    E. melis
    E. paryphostomum
    E. perfoliatum
    E. revolutum
echinostomiasis
ECHO virus (enteric cytopathogenic human orphan virus)
ECHO virus
    type 1
    type 12
ECHO 28 virus
ECI (electrocerebral inactivity)

Additional Entries

eclampsia
    puerperal e.
    uremic e.
ECM (erythema chronicum migrans)
ECMO virus (enteric cytopathogenic monkey orphan virus)
E. coli (Escherichia coli)
Economo's disease
ECSO virus (enteric cytopathogenic swine orphan virus)
ectasia
    mammary duct e.
ecthyma
    e. gangrenosum
    e. infectiosum
ectodermal dysplasia
ectoparasite
ectopia
ectopic
    e. anus
    e. hormone
    e. pregnancy
    e. tissue
ectromelia
ectromelus
ectrometacarpia
ectylurea
eczema
    e. herpeticum
    mummular e.
eczematoid dermatitis
ED (Ehlers-Danlos syndrome, epileptiform discharge)
Eddowes's disease
edema

edema *(continued)*
    angioneurotic e.
    cerebral e.
    peripheral e.
    pulmonary e.
EDS (Ehlers-Danlos syndrome)
Edsall's disease
Edwardsiella
    E. tarda
Edwardsielleae
Edwards-Patau syndrome
EEC (Escherichia coli)
EEE (eastern equine encephalomyelitis)
EEE virus (eastern equine encephalomyelitis virus)
eelworm
EFE (endocardial fibroelastosis)
effect
effusion
    chylous e.
    serofibrinous e.
    serosanguineous e.
    serous e.
EGL (eosinophilic granuloma of the lung)
EH (essential hypertension)
EHBF (exercise hyperemia blood flow)
EHC (essential hypercholesterolemia)
EHF (exophthalmos-hyperthyroid factor)
EHL (endogenous hyperlipidemia)
Ehlers-Danlos syndrome
EHO (extrahepatic obstruction)
EHP (excessive heat production)

Additional Entries

Eichstedt's disease
Eikenella
    E. corrodens
Eisenlohr's syndrome
Eisenmenger's syndrome
Ekbom syndrome
EKC (epidemic keratoconjunctivitis)
elastofibroma
    e. dorsi
elastosis
    e. perforans serpiginosa
    senile e.
elephantiasis
    e. nostras
elliptocytosis
    hereditary e.
Ellis-van Creveld syndrome
Em (emmetropia)
emaciation
Embadomonas
embolic
    e. aneurysm
    e. glomerulonephritis
embolism
    air e.
    amniotic fluid e.
    arterial e.
    bacillary e.
    bone-marrow e.
    capillary e.
    cerebral e.
    coronary e.
    fat e.
    gas e.
    infective e.
    lymph e.
    miliary e.

embolism *(continued)*
    paradoxical e.
    plasmodium e.
    pulmonary e.
    pyemic e.
    retinal e.
    saddle e.
    spinal e.
    trichinous e.
    venous e.
embolus (emboli)
    air e.
    amniotic fluid e.
    atheromatous e.
    bland e.
    bone marrow e.
    fat e.
    foreign body e.
    massive e.
    paradoxical e.
    parasitic e.
    recent e.
    eptic e.
    tumor e.
    valvular tissue e.
embryo
    nodular e.
    stunted e.
embryoma
embryonal
    e. adenoma
    e. carcinoma
    e. cell carcinoma
    e. duct cyst
    e. nephroma
    e. rhabdomyosarcoma
    e. teratoma
EMC (encephalomyocarditis)

Additional Entries

EMC virus
    (encephalomyocarditis virus)
emesis
EMF (endomyocardial fibrosis)
EMG (exophthalmos, macroglossia, gigantism)
Emmonsia
Emmonsiella
emperipolesis
emphraxis
emphysema
    bullous e.
    centrilobular e.
    compensatory e.
    interstitial e.
    obstructive e.
    panacinar e.
    pulmonary e.
    subcutaneous e.
    vesicular e.
emphysematous
    e. bleb
    e. vaginitis
empty sella syndrome
empyema
    subdural e.
EN (erythema nodosum)
enamel
    e. hypoplasia
    mottled e.
enamelogenesis imperfecta
encephalitis
    arthropod-borne virus e.
    California e.
    eastern equine e.
    e. herpes simplex
    e. lethargica
    post-infectious allergic e.

encephalitis *(continued)*
    post-vaccination allergic e.
    St. Louis e.
    Venezuelan equine e.
    western e.
encephalocystocele
encephalomalacia
encephalomeningocele
encephalomyelitis
    autoimmune e.
encephalomyelopathy
encephalomyocarditis
encephalopathy
    anoxic e.
    hepatic e.
    hypercapnic e.
    hypertensive e.
    hypoglycemic e.
    lead e.
    uremic e.
    Wernicke's e.
encephalotrigeminal angiomatosis
enchondroma
enchondrosarcoma
enchondrosis
Endamoeba
    E. blattae
endarteritis
    e. obliterans
endemic
    e. goiter
    e. hemoptysis
    e. typhus
endocardial
    e. fibroelastosis
    e. sclerosis

Additional Entries

endocardiosis
    nonbacterial verrucal e.
endocarditis
    atypical verrucal e.
    bacterial e.
    Libman-Sacks e.
    marantic e.
    nonbacterial thrombotic e.
    rheumatic e.
    vegetative e.
    verrucous e.
endocervicitis
endocrine
    e. adenomatosis
endocrinopathy
endocytosis
endodermal
    e. sinus tumor
Endodermophyton
endogenous
    e. hemosiderosis
Endolimax
    E. nana
endolymphatic
    e. stromal myosis
endometrial
    e. atrophy
    e. hyperplasia
    e. polyp
    e. stroma
    e. stromal sarcoma
    e. stromatosis
endometrioma
endometriosis
    stromal e.
endometritis
    syncytial e.
endometrium

endometrium *(continued)*
    atrophic e.
    inactive e.
    senile e.
endomitosis
Endomyces
    E. albicans
    E. capsulatus
    E. epidermatidis
    E. epidermidis
endomycosis
endomyocardial
    e. fibrosis
    e. sclerosis
endoparasite
endophlebitis
endophthalmitis
endophlebitis
endopolyploidy
endothelial
    e. metaplasia
    e. sarcoma
endothelioma
endotoxemia
endotoxic shock
Engelmann's disease
Engel-Recklinghausen disease
English disease
Engman's disease
ENL (erythema nodosum leproticum)
enostosis
entamebiasis
Entamoeba
    E. buccalis
    E. buetschlii
    E. coli
    E. gingivalis

Additional Entries

Entamoeba *(continued)*
    E. hartmanni
    E. histolytica
    E. nana
    E. nipponica
    E. polecki
    E. tetragena
    E. tropicalis
enteric
    e. cytopathogenic human orphan virus
Enteritidis
    E. salmonella
enteritis
    regional e.
    staphylococcal e.
Enterobacter
    E. aerogenes
    E. agglomerans
    E. alvei
    E. cloacae
    E. gergoviae
    E. hafniae
    E. liquefaciens
    E. sakazakii
    E. subgroup C.
Enterobacteriaceae
enterobiasis
Enterobius
    E. vermicularis
enterocele
enterocolitis
    acute necrotizing e.
    cicatrizing e.
    pseudomembranous e.
    regional e.
enterolith
Enteromonas

Enteromonas *(continued)*
    E. hominis
enteropathy
    gluten-sensitive e.
    protein-losing e.
enterotoxigenic
enterotoxin
enterovirus
Entoloma lividum
Entomophthora
    E. coronata
entomophthoromycosis
enuresis
environmental stress
enzymic fat necrosis
eosinopenia
eosinophil
    e. adenoma
    e. chemotactic factor of anaphylaxis
eosinophilic
    e. fasciitis
    e. granuloma
    e. hyperplasia
    e. leukemia
EP (ectopic pregnancy)
EPC (epilepsia partialis continua)
EPEC (enteropathogenic Escherichia coli)
ependymoblastoma
ependymoma
    epithelial e.
    Grade I e.
    Grades II - IV e.
    malignant e.
    myxopapillary e.
    papillary e.

Additional Entries
___
___
___
___
___

EPF (exophthalmos-producing
  factor)
epicanthus
epicarcinogen
epicondylitis
epidemic
  hemorrhagic fever e.
  parotitis virus e.
  typhus e.
epidermal
  e. cyst
  e. dermal nevus
  e. inclusion cyst
epidermodysplasia
  e. verruciformis
epidermoid
  e. carcinoma
  e. carcinoma-in-situ
  e. cyst
  e. inclusion cyst
  e. metaplasia
epidermolysis
  e. bullosa
Epidermophyton
  E. floccosum
  E. inguinale
  E. rubrum
epidermophytosis
epididymitis
epidural
  e. hematoma
epigastrius parasiticus
epilepsy
  familial myoclonic e.
  focal e.
  focal cortical e.
  grand mal e.
  jacksonian e.

epilepsy *(continued)*
  minor e.
  myoclonic e.
  petit mal e.
  post-traumatic e.
  psychomotor e.
  rolandic e.
  temporal lobe e.
  uncinate e.
epileptiform
epiphyseal
  e. giant cell tumor
episcleritis
  rheumatoid e.
epistasis
epistaxis
epithelial
  e. cyst
  e. ependymoma
  e. hyperplasia
  e. inclusion cyst
  e. neoplasm
  e. tumor
epithelioid
  e. cell melanoma
  e. cell nevus
  e. sarcoma
epithelioma
  e. adenoides cysticum
  basal cell e.
  benign e.
  Borst-Jadassohn
    intraepidermal basal
    cell e.
  Malherbe's calcifying e.
epitheliosis
EPS (exophthalmos-producing
  substance)

Additional Entries

Epstein-Barr virus
equine encephalitis
    eastern e. e.
    Venezuelan e. e.
    western e. e.
Erb-Charcot disease
Erb-Goldflam disease
Erb-Landouzy disease
Erb's palsy
Erdheim disease
erosive
    e. aneurysm
    e. esophagitis
    e. gastritis
    e. inflammation
ERP (equine rhinopneumonitis)
eructation
eruption
    bullous e.
    Kaposi's varicelliform e.
    macular e.
    maculopapular e.
    polymorphic light e.
    polymorphous e.
Erwinia
    E. amylovora
    E. herbicola
Erysipelothrix
    E. insidiosa
    E. rhusiopathiae
erythema
    e. ab igne
    e. annular centrifugum
    e. chronicum migrans
    e. figuratum
    e. induratum
    e. infectiosum

erythema *(continued)*
    e. marginatum rheumaticum
    e. multiforme
    e. multiforme exudativum
    e. neonatorum
    e. nodosum
    Osler's e.
    palmar e.
    e. pernio
    e. perstans
    toxic e.
erythrasma
erythremia
erythremic myelosis
Erythrobacillus
erythroblastomatosis
erythroblastosis
    e. fetalis
    e. neonatorum
erythrocythemia
erythrocytosis
    leukemic e.
    e. megalosplenica
erythrodontia
erythroid
    e. aplasia
    e. hyperplasia
    e. hypoplasia
erythroleukemia
erythromyeloblastic leukemia
erythroneocytosis
erythropenia
erythrophagocytosis
erythroplasia
    Queyrat's e.
Escherichia
    E. aerogenes

Additional Entries

Escherichia *(continued)*
    E. alkalescens
    E. aurescens
    E. coli
    E. dispar
    E. dispar var. ceylonensis
    E. dispar var. madampensis
    E. freundii
    E. intermedia
Escherichieae
Escherich's bacillus
ESM (ejection systolic murmur)
esophageal
    e. achalasia
    e. varices
esophagitis
    corrosive e.
    erosive e.
    infectious e.
    monilial e.
    peptic e.
    reflux e.
esophagomalacia
esophagus
    Barrett's e.
essential
    e. atrophy
    e. hypercholesterolemia
    e. hyperlipemia
    e. hypertension
    e. pentosuria
esthesioneurocytoma
Estren-Dameshek anemia
etiology
    genetic e.
    unknown e.
eubacteria

Eubacterium
    E. aerofaciens
    E. alactolyticum
    E. contortum
    E. endocarditis
    E. lentum
    E. limosum
    E. parvum
    E. rectale
    E. ventriosum
Euglena
    E. gracilis
eukaryosis
Eulenburg's disease
Euproctis
    E. chrysorrhoea
European
    E. blastomycosis
    E. hookworm
    E. rat flea
Eurotium
    E. malignum
Eustrogylus
euthyroidism
Eutriatoma
Eutrombicula
    E. alfreddugesi
evisceration
Ewing's
    sarcoma
    tumor
ex (exophthalmos)
exanthem
    Boston e.
    e. subitum
exanthematous
excessive
    e. cornification

Additional Entries

excessive *(continued)*
    e. fatigue
    e. lacrimation
    e. sweating
    e. tearing
    e. weakness
    e. weeping
    e. weight gain
    e. weight loss
excoriation
excretion
    pseudouridine e.
exertional dyspnea
exfoliation
exfoliative
    e. cytologic alteration
    e. dermatitis
    e. psoriasis
exhaustion
    e. atrophy
    heat e.
exocytosis

exogenous
    e. obesity
    e. hemosiderosis
Exophiala
    E. jeanselmei
    E. mycetoma
    E. werneckii
exophthalmos
exostosis
    cartilaginous e.
    osteocartilaginous e.
exothermic
exotoxin
external
    e. endometriosis
    e. hemorrhoids
    e. hydrocephalus
extramammary Paget's disease
extrauterine pregnancy
exudate
    acute inflammatory e.

Additional Entries

F

F. (Filaria, Fusiformis)
Faber's syndrome
Fabry's disease
face
    adenoid f.
    cleft f.
facet syndrome
facial
    f. myiasis
    f. palsy
facies
    f. abdominalis
    adenoid f.
    cushingoid f.
    f. hepatica
    f. hippocratica
    f. leontina
    leprechaun f.
    Parkinson's f.
    scaphoid f.
facioplegic
    f. migraine
facioscapulohumeral-type progressive muscular dystrophy
factitious
    f. dermatitis
    f. urticaria
falciparum malaria
false
    f. aneurysm
    f. diverticulum
    f. hernia
    f. knot umbilical cord
    f. negative

false *(continued)*
    f. positive
familial
    f. benign pemphigus Hailey-Hailey disease
    f. cardiomyopathy
    f. cerebellar ataxia
    f. erythrophagocytic lymphohistiocytosis
    f. fibrous dysplasia
    f. gonadal dysgenesis
    f. hemolytic anemia
    f. hypercholesterolemia
    f. Mediterranean fever
    f. myoclonic epilepsy
    f. nephritis
    f. nephronophthisis
    f. nonhemolytic jaundice
    f. periodic paralysis
    f. polyposis
    f. primary systemic amyloidosis
Fanconi's
    anemia
    syndrome
Fanconi-Zinssen syndrome
Fannia
    F. canicularis
    F. scalaris
Farber's
    disease
    lipogranulomatosis
farmer's lung
fascial fibrosarcoma
fasciitis

Additional Entries

fasciitis *(continued)*
    eosinophilic f.
    infiltrative f.
    necrotizing f.
    nodular f.
    pseudosarcomatous f.
Fasciola
    F. gigantica
    F. hepatica
fascioliasis
fasciolopsiasis
Fasciolopsis
    F. buski
fat
    f. embolism
    f. embolus
    f. necrosis
fatigue
fatty
    f. atrophy
    f. degeneration
    f. nutritional cirrhosis
    f. phanerosis
FAV (feline ataxia virus)
FD (fatal dose)
febrile
fecal
    f. impaction
    f. incontinence
    f. vomitus
fecalith
feces
    extravasation f.
    impacted f.
Fehleisen's streptococcus
FEL (familial erythrophagocytic lymphohistiocytosis)
Felty's syndrome

feminization
    f. syndrome, adrenal
    testicular f.
feminizing tumor
femorocele
fenestration
    atrophic f.
Ferribacterium
ferrocalcinosis
ferrocalcinotic deposition
fetal
    f. abnormality
    f. adenoma
    f. fat cell lipoma
    f. lipoma
fetid rhinitis
fetus
    f. acardiacus
    f. amorphus
    f. compressus
    f. in fetu
    macerated f.
    f. papyraceus
    parasitic f.
    stunted f.
fever
    Bullis f.
    Bwamba f.
    chikungunya f.
    Colorado f.
    Dumdum f.
    familial Mediterranean f.
    Haverhill f.
    Malta f.
    Mediterranean f.
    Omsk hemorrhagic f.
    O'nyong-nyong f.
    Oroya f.

Additional Entries

fever *(continued)*
    pappataci f.
    Pel-Ebstein f.
    Pontiac f.
    Q. f.
    Rocky Mountain spotted f.
    San Joaquin f.
    undulant f.
    West Nile f.
FGD (fatal granulomatous disease)
FI (fever caused by infection)
fibrillary astrocytoma
fibrillation
    atrial f.
    auricular f.
    cardiac f.
    muscular f.
    ventricular f.
fibrinogen deficiency
fibrinogenopenia
fibrinoid
    f. necrosis
    f. necrotizing inflammation
fibrinolytic purpura
fibrinopenia
fibrinopurulent
fibrinous
    f. acute lobar pneumonia
    f. acute pleuritis
    f. adhesion
    f. exudation
    f. inflammation
    f. peritonitis
    f. pleurisy
    f. pleuritis
fibroadenoma

fibroadenoma *(continued)*
    giant f.
    intracanalicular f.
    juvenile f.
    pericanalicular f.
fibroadenosis
fibroameloblastic
    f. dentinoma
    f. odontoma
fibroblastic meningioma
fibroblastoma
    perineural f.
fibrocalcific
fibrocongestive
    f. hypertrophy
    f. splenomegaly
fibrocystic
    f. disease, breast
    f. mastitis
    f. mastopathy
fibroelastosis
    endocardial f.
fibroepithelial
    f. papilloma
    f. polyp
fibroepithelioma
fibrogenesis
    f. imperfecta ossium
fibroid uterus
fibrolipoma
fibroliposarcoma
fibroma
    ameloblastic f.
    cementifying f.
    chondromyxoid f.
    myxoid f.
    nonossifying f.
    odontogenic f.

Additional Entries

fibroma *(continued)*
    ossifying f.
    periosteal f.
    peripheral odontogenic f.
fibromatosis
    f. colli
    Dupuytren's f.
    palmar f.
    plantar f.
fibromyoma
fibromyositis
fibromyxoid
fibromyxolipoma
fibromyxoma
fibromyxosarcoma
fibroplasia
    retrolental f.
fibrosarcoma
    fascial f.
    medullary f.
    odontogenic f.
    periosteal f.
fibrosiderotic nodule
fibrosing
    f. adenomatosis
    f. adenosis
    f. alveolitis
    condensation f.
    cystic f.
    diffuse f.
    endomyocardial f.
    focal f.
    hepatic f.
    inflammation with f.
    interstitial f.
    mediastinal f.
    multifocal f.
    nodular f.

fibrosing *(continued)*
    pulmonary f.
    retroperitoneal f.
    septal f
    subepidermal f.
fibrotic
fibrous
    f. adhesion
    f ankylosis
    f. astrocytoma
    f. cortical defect
    f. dysplasia
    f. histiocytoma
    f. hypertrophic pachymeningitis
    f. mesothelioma
    f. nodule
    f. osteoma
    f. thyroiditis
fibroxanthoma
Fick's bacillus
Fielder's myocarditis
Filaria
    F. bancrofti
    F. conjunctivae
    F. demarquayi
    F. hominis oris
    F. juncea
    F. labialis
    F. lentis
    F. loa
    F. lymphatica
    F. medinensis
    F. ozzardi
    F. palpebralis
    F. philippinensis
    F. sanguinis
    F. tucumana

Additional Entries

Filaria *(continued)*
    F. volvulus
filariasis
    Bancroft's f.
    Malayan f.
filiform
    f. hyperkeratosis
filling
    f. defect
    f. gallop
    f. rumble
Filobasidiella
    F. bacillisporus
    F. neoformans
first degree
    f. d. burn
    f. d. frostbite
    f. d. heart block
    f. d. radiation injury
fistula
FJN (familial juvenile nephrophthisis)
flaccid
flatulence
flatworm
flavivirus
Flavobacterium
    F. meningosepticum
flea
    American rat f.
    dog f.
    European rat f.
    human f.
    Indian rat f.
Flexner's
    bacillus
    dysentery
Flexner-Strong bacillus

floccular degeneration
floppy valve syndrome
FLSA (follicular lymphosarcoma)
flu (influenza)
fluke
    blood f.
    cat liver f.
    Chinese liver f.
    giant intestinal f.
    giant liver f.
    liver f.
    oriental lung f.
    sheep liver f.
    Yokogawa's f.
flutter
    atrial f.
    ventricular f.
fly
    black f.
    bot f.
    deer f.
    horse f.
    house f.
    larval f.
    stable f.
    tsetse f.
    warble f.
FMF (familial Mediterranean fever)
FN (false negative)
FOAVF (failure of all vital forces)
focal
    f. epilepsy
    f. segmental glomerulosclerosis
folate

Additional Entries

folate *(continued)*
   f. deficiency anemia
follicle
   atretic f.
   cyst f.
   cystic ovarian f.
follicular
   f. adenocarcinoma
   f. adenoma
   f. carcinoma
   f. conjunctivitis
   f. cyst
   f. dermatitis
   f. inflammation
   f. inverted keratosis
   f. lymphoma
   f. and papillary
     adenocarcinoma
   f. salpingitis
   f. urethritis
folliculitis
   f. decalvans
   f. keloidalis
   f. ulerythematosa
     reticulata
Fonsecaea
   F. compactum
   F. dermatitidis
   F. jeanselmei
   F. pedrosoi
food
   f. deprevation
   f. intolerance
   f. poisoning
foot-and-mouth disease
foot-and-mouth disease virus,
   types A, B, C
Forbe's disease

Fordyce's disease
fourth degree
   f. d. burn
   f. d. frostbite
   f. d. radiation injury
Fox-Fordyce disease
FP (false positive)
fracture
   chip f.
   closed f.
   comminuted f.
   compressed f.
   depressed f.
   f. dislocation
   greenstick f.
   healed f.
   impacted f.
   incomplete f.
   linear f.
   nonunion f.
   oblique f.
   pathologic f.
   simple f.
   spiral f.
   stellate f.
   transverse f.
   ununited f.
fragmentation
   f. of myocardium
frambesia
Francisella
   F. tularensis
Franklin's disease
freckle
   Hutchinson's melanotic f.
freezing injury
friction rub
   pericardial f. r.

Additional Entries

friction rub *(continued)*
    pleural f. r.
Friedlander's
    bacillus
    pneumobacillus
    pneumonia
Friedreich's ataxia
frigidity
Frohlich's syndrome
Frommel-Chiari syndrome
frostbite
fructosemia
fructosuria
fucosidosis
fungus
    ascospore-forming f.
    cutaneous f.
    fission f.
    mosaic f.
    mycelial f.
    yeast f.
funnel chest
FUO (fever of undetermined origin)
furunculosis
fusariomycosis
Fusarium
    F. javanicum
    F. moniliforme

Fusarium *(continued)*
    F. oxysporum
    F. roseum
    F. solanae
    F. sporotrichoides
Fusidum terricola
fusiform
    f. aneurysm
    f. bronchiectasis
Fusiformis
    F. necrophorus
Fusobacterium
    F. aquatile
    F. fusiforme
    F. glutinosum
    F. gonidiaformans
    F. mortiferum
    F. naviforme
    F. necrophorum
    F. nucleatum
    F. plautivincenti
    F. prausnitzii
    F. symbiosum
    F. varium
fusospirillosis
fusospirochetal
fusospirochetosis
fusostreptococcicosis

Additional Entries

Additional Entries

G

Gaffkya
    G. tetragena
Gaisbock's disease
gait
    athetotic g.
    choreic g.
    g. disturbance
    dystonic g.
    festinating g.
    reeling g.
    shuffling g.
    spastic g.
    staggering g.
    steppage g.
    g. unsteadiness
    waddling g.
galactocele
galactorrhea
galactosemia
galactosuria
galacturia
Galerina
    G. autumnalis
    G. marginata
    G. venerata
gametocytemia
gamma
    g. heavy chain disease
    g. streptococcus
gammaglobulinopathy
gammopathy
    monoclonal g.
    polyclonal g.
ganglioglioma
ganglion

ganglion *(continued)*
    g. cyst
ganglioneuroblastoma
ganglioneuroma
gangliosidosis
    generalized g.
    GM(SB)1 g.
    GM(SB)2 g.
gangosa
gangrene
    dry g.
    gas g.
    progressive bacterial
        synergistic g.
    static g.
    trophic g.
    venous g.
gangrenous
    g. appendicitis
    g. inflammation
    g. necrosis
Ganser's syndrome
Gardnerella vaginalis
Gardner's syndrome
gargoylism
Garre's sclerosing osteomyelitis
Gartner's
    bacillus
    duct cyst
gas
    g. embolism
    g. extravasation
    g. gangrene
    g. retention
gaseous

Additional Entries

Gasteromycetes
Gasterophilus
gastric
    g. atrophy
    g. myiasis
    g. ulcer, perforated
    g. vomitus
gastrinoma
gastritis
    acute g.
    antral g.
    atrophic g.
    chronic atrophic g.
    chronic hypertrophic g.
    erosive g.
    giant hypertrophic g.
    hemorrhagic g.
    hypertrophic g.
    phlegmonous g.
gastrocele
gastrocolic
gastrodisciasis
Gastrodiscoides
    G. hominis
Gastrodiscus
    G. hominis
gastroenteritis
gastroenteropathy
gastroenteroptosis
gastrointestinal
    g. fistula
gastrojejunal
    g. fistula
gastromalacia
gastroparesis
gastrophthisis
gastrosia fungosa
Gaucher's disease

GB (Guillain-Barre syndrome)
GC (gonococcus, gonorrhea)
Gee-Herter-Heubner disease
Gee-Thaysen disease
gelatinous
    g. acute inflammation
    g. acute pneumonia
    g. adenocarcinoma
    g. atrophy
    g. carcinoma
    g. inflammation
gemistocytic
    g. astrocytoma
    g. tumor
genitourinary
    g. myiasis
Geodermatophilus
geophagia
geotrichosis
Geotrichum
    G. candidum
    G. immite
German measles virus
germinoma
    pineal g.
geroderma
    g. osteodysplastica
gestational
    g. alteration
    g. trophoblastic disease
gestosis
Ghon-Sachs bacillus
giant
    g. blue nevus
    g. fibroadenoma
    g. follicle lymphoma
    g. hairy nevus
    g. intestinal fluke

Additional Entries

giant *(continued)*
    g. intracanalicular
        fibroadenoma
    g. neutrophilia
    g. osteoid osteoma
    g. rugal hypertrophy
    g. urticaria
giant cell
    g. c. arteritis
    g. c. carcinoma
    g. c. granuloma
    g. c. hepatitis
    g. c. myocarditis
    g. c. pneumonia
    g. c. sarcoma
    g. c. thyroiditis
    g. c. tumor
giantism
Giardia
    G. intestinalis
    G. lamblia
giardiasis
Gibberella fujikuroi
gibbon ape lymphosarcoma
    virus
Gierke's disease
gigantism
gigantomastia
Gilbert's syndrome
Gilchrist's disease
Gilles de la Tourette's syndrome
gingival
    g. hyperplasia
gingivitis
    diphenylhydantoin g.
    hypertrophic g.
    scorbutic g.
gingivosis

gingivostomatitis
    herpetic g.
    necrotizing ulcerative g.
glandular
    g. metaplasia
Glanzmann-Naegeli
    thrombasthenia
Glanzmann's thrombasthenia
glassy
    g. cell carcinoma
glaucoma
    angle closure g.
    congenital g.
    infantile g.
    open angle g.
    primary g.
    secondary g.
Glenospora graphii
Glenosporella loboi
glioblastoma multiforme
Gliocladium
glioma
    malignant g.
    mixed g.
    nasal g.
    subependymal g.
gliomatosis
gliosarcoma
gliosis
gliotoxin
globoid leukodystrophy
globulinuria
globulomaxillary cyst
glomangioma
glomerulitis
glomerulonephritis
    acute g.
    acute exudative g.

Additional Entries

glomerulonephritis *(continued)*
    acute hemorrhagic g.
    antibasement membrane g.
    chronic g.
    diffuse g.
    embolic g.
    exudative g.
    focal g.
    hemorrhagic g.
    lobular g.
    membranous g.
    mesangial proliferative g.
    necrotizing g.
    proliferative g.
    rapidly progressive g.
    subacute g.
glomerulopathy
glomerulosclerosis
    cirrhotic g.
    diabetic g.
    intercapillary g.
    nodular g.
Glossina
glossitis
    Hunter's g.
    median rhomboid g.
glossopharyngeal neuralgia
glucagonoma
glucatonia
glutathionemia
glutathionuria
gluten
    g.-sensitive enteropathy
glycinemia
glycinuria
Glyciphagus
    G. buski
    G. domesticus

glycogen storage disease
glycogenesis
    hepatophosphorylase deficiency g.
    hepatorenal, glucose-6-phosphatase deficiency g.
    idiopathic generalized g.
    myophosphorylase deficiency g.
glycosuria
    pathologic g.
    renal g.
    toxic g.
glycosuric
    g. melituria
Glycyphagus
    G. domesticus
Gnathostoma
    G. hispidum
    G. spinigerum
gnathostomiasis
goiter
    adenomatous g.
    colloid g.
    congenital g.
    diffuse g.
    dyshormonogenic g.
    endemic g.
    exophthalmic g.
    hyperplastic g.
    lymphadenoid g.
    multinodular g.
    nodular g.
    parenchymatous g.
    simple g.
    sporadic diffuse g.
    sporadic nodular g.

Additional Entries

goiter *(continued)*
    substernal g.
    toxic g.
Goldblatt's
    hypertension
    kidney
Goldflam's disease
gonadal
    g. dysgenesis
    g. endocrine disorder
    g. stromal tumor
Gongylonema pulchrum
gongylonemiasis
gonococcal arthritis-dermatitis
    sydrome
gonococcus
gonorrhea
Goodell's sign
Goodpasture's syndrome
Good's syndrome
Gordius
    G. aquaticus
    G. robustus
Gorham's disease
gout
GP (general paresis)
grain
    g. itch
    g. itch mite
gram-negative
    bacilli
    bacteria
    cocci
gram-positive
    bacilli
    bacteria
    cocci
grand mal

granular
    g. atrophy
    g. cell myoblastoma
    g. cell tumor
    g. degeneration
    g. urethritis
granuloblastosis
granulocytic
    g. aplasia
    g. hyperplasia
    g. hypoplasia
    g. leukemia
granulocytopenia
granulocytosis
granuloma
    g. annulare
    apical g.
    beryllium g.
    calcified g.
    caseating g.
    dental g.
    eosinophilic g.
    g. faciale
    foreign body g.
    giant cell reparative g.
    histiocytic g.
    Hodgkin's g.
    g. inguinale
    lethal midline g.
    lipoid g.
    Majocchi's g.
    mineral oil g.
    multifocal eosinophilic g.
    non-necrotizing g.
    plasma cell g.
    pyogenic g.
    reticulohistiocytic g.
    sarcoid g.

Additional Entries

granuloma *(continued)*
    spermatogenic g.
    suture g.
    swimming pool g.
    tuberculoid g.
    unifocal eosinophilic g.
granulomatosis
    allergic g.
    angiitic g.
    Wegener's g
granulomatous
    g. colitis
    g. inflammation
    g. polyp
    g. thyroiditis
granulopenia
granulophthisis
granulosa cell
    g. c. carcinoma
    g. c. theca cell tumor
    g. c. tumor
Grave's disease
Grawitz's tumor
gray
    g.-patch ringworm
    g. platelet syndrome
    g. scale
GU (gastric ulcer, gonococcal urethritis)
Guama virus
guanidinemia
Guaroa virus
Guillain-Barre syndrome
Gull's disease
Gymnoascus
gymnobacterium
gynecomastia

Additional Entries

H

H (hypermetropia)
    H. (Hemophilus)
HA (hemolytic anemia)
HAA (hepatitis-associated antigen)
Haemagogus
Haemaphysalis
    H. concinna
    H. leporispalustris
    H. spinigera
Haemonchus
    H. contortus
    H. placei
Haemophilus (Hemophilus)
Hafnia alvei
Hailey-Hailey disease
Hallervorden-Spatz disease
hamartoma
Hamman-Rich syndrome
Hamman's disease
hammer toe
Hand-Schuller-Christian disease
Hansen's
    bacillus
    disease
Hansenula
HAP (heredopathia atactica polyneuritiformis)
hapalonychia
Harada's syndrome
Hartmanella
    H. hyalina
Hartnup disease
Hashimoto's
    disease

Hashimoto's *(continued)*
    struma
    thyroiditis
HAV (hepatitis A virus)
Haverhillia
    H. moniliformis
    H. multiformis
hay fever
HB (hepatitis B, heart block)
HBV (hepatitis B virus)
HC (Huntington's chorea)
HCVD (hypertensive cardiovascular disease)
HD (heart disease, Hodgkin's disease, hydatid disease)
HE (hereditary elliptocytosis)
heart
    h. block
    h. disease
    h. failure
    hypoplastic h.
heartburn
heartworm
heavy chain disease
hebephrenic schizophrenia
Heerfordt's disease
Heinz body hemolytic anemia
helminthiasis
helminthic
Helminthosporium
Helophilus
Helvella
    H. esculenta
hemangioblastoma
hemangioendothelial sarcoma

Additional Entries

hemangioendothelioma
hemangiolipoma
hemangioma
    ameloblastic h.
    capillary h.
    cavernous h.
    infantile h.
    sclerosing h.
hemangiomatosis
hemangiopericytoma
hemangiosarcoma
hemapheresis
hemarthrosis
hematemesis
hematidrosis
hematocele
hematochezia
hematoclasis
hematoclastic
hematoma
    epidural h.
    subdural h.
hematometra
hematopoietic
    h. aplasia
    h. cell cytoplasmic
      alteration
    h. hyperplasia
hematuria
hemianalgesia
hemianesthesia
hemianopia
hemianopsia
    binasal h.
    bitemporal h
    homonymous h.
hemiatrophy
hemiblock

hemimelia
hemiparesis
hemiplegia
Hemispora stellata
hemochromatosis
hemocystinuria
hemoglobinemia
hemoglobinopathy
    heterozygous h.
    homozygous h.
    mixed h.
hemoglobinorrhea
hemoglobinuria
    bacillary h.
    epidemic h.
    malarial h.
    march h.
    paroxysmal h.
    paroxysmal cold h.
    paroxysmal nocturnal h.
    toxic h.
hemoglobinuric
    h. nephrosis
hemokinesis
hemolysis
hemolytic
    h. anemia
    h. disease of the newborn
    h. jaundice
hemophilia
    h. A
    h. B
    h. C
    vascular h.
hemophiliac
hemophilic
Hemophilus
    H. aegyptius

Additional Entries

Hemophilus *(continued)*
   H. aphrophilus
   H. bronchisepticus
   H. conjunctivitidis
   H. ducreyi
   H. duplex
   H. hemoglobinophilus
   H. hemolyticus
   H. influenzae
   H. parahemolyticus
   H. parainfluenzae
   H. parapertussis
   H. paraphrohemolyticus
   H. paraphrophilus
   H. pertussis
   H. suis
   H. vaginalis
hemophilus
   h. of Koch-Weeks
   h. of Morax-Axenfeld
hemophthalmia
hemopneumopericardium
hemopneumothorax
hemoptysis
   cardiac h.
   oriental h.
   parasitic h.
   vicarious h.
hemorrhage
   petechial h.
hemorrhagic
   acute h. bronchopneumonia
   acute h. cholecystitis
   acute h. cystitis
   acute h. glomerulonephritis
   acute h. inflammation

hemorrhagic *(continued)*
   acute h. ulcer
   acute h. ulceration
   h. ascites
   h. bronchopneumonia
   h. cyst
   h. cystitis
   h. disease of the newborn
   h. diverticulitis
   h. fever
   h. gastritis
   h. glomerulonephritis
   h. infarct
   h. inflammation
   h. lobar pneumonia
   h. shock
   h. thrombocythemia
   h. ulcer
hemorrhoid
   thrombosed h.
hemorrhoidal
   h. artery
   h. nerve
   h. vein
   h. zone
hemosiderinuria
hemosiderosis
   endogenous h.
   exogenous h.
   idiopathic pulmonary h.
Henoch-Schonlein syndrome
Henoch's purpura
hepatic encephalopathy
hepatitis
   acute focal h.
   A virus h.
   B virus h.
   giant cell h.

Additional Entries

hepatitis *(continued)*
    infectious h.
    serum h.
    viral h.
hepatocele
hepatocellular
    h. carcinoma
    h. jaundice
hepatocholangitis
hepatolenticular degeneration
hepatoma
hepatomegaly
hepatophosphorylase deficiency
hepatorenal syndrome
hepatosplenomegaly
hereditary spherocytosis
Herellea
    H. vaginicola
Hermansky-Pudlak syndrome
Hermetia illucens
hernia
    diaphragmatic h.
    epigastric h.
    esophageal h.
    femoral h.
    hiatal h.
    incarcerated h.
    inguinal h.
    irreducible h.
    Morgagni's h.
    peritoneal h.
    retrocolic h.
    retrosternal h.
    Richter's h.
    strangulated h.
    umbilical h.
herniated
    h. nucleus pulposus

herpes
    h. corneae
    h. febrilis
    h. genitalis
    h. gestationis
    h. simplex
    h. simplex virus, I, II
    h. zoster
    h. zoster virus
herpesvirus
Herpetomonas
Hers' disease
heterauxesis
Heterobilharzia
Heterodera
    H. marioni
    H. radicicola
Heterophyes
    H. heterophyes
    H. katsuradai
Heterophyes/Metagonimus
heterophyiasis
heteropyknotic
heterosis
heterosomal
    h. aberration
heterothallism
heterotopia
heterotopic
heterozygous
    h. hemoglobinopathy
    h. thalassemia
    h. type of hemoglobin disorder
HF (hay fever, heart failure, hemorrhagic fever)
HFI (hereditary fructose intolerance)

Additional Entries

HHA (hereditary hemolytic anemia)
HHD (hypertensive heart disease)
H and Hm (compound hypermetropic astigmatism)
HHT (hereditary hemorrhagic telangiectasia)
hiatus hernia
hibernoma
hidradenitis suppurativa
hidradenoma
    clear cell h.
    nodular h.
    papillary h.
hidrocystoma
high frequency deafness
hilar cell tumor
Hippel-Lindau disease
Hippel's disease
hippuria
Hirschsprung's disease
hirsutism
hirudiniasis
Hirudo
    H. aegyptiaca
    H. medicinalis
histidinemia
histidinuria
histiocytic
    h. granuloma
    h. leukemia
    h. lymphoma
    h. reticulosis, medullary
histiocytoma
histiocytosis
    kerasin-type h.
    lipid h.

histiocytosis *(continued)*
    nonlipid h.
    phosphatid-type h.
    h. X
histopathology
Histoplasma
    H. capsulatum
    H. duboisii
    H. farciminosus
histoplasmosis
HIT (hypertrophic infiltrative tendinitis)
HL (histiocytic lymphoma; hypermetropic, latent)
HLV (herpes-like virus)
HM (hydatidiform mole)
Hm (manifest hyperopia)
HMD (hyaline membrane disease)
HMSAS (hypertrophic muscular subaortic stenosis)
HN (hereditary nephritis)
HNP (herniated nucleus pulposus)
HNSHA (hereditary nonspherocytic hemolytic anemia)
HOCM (hypertrophic obstructive cardiomyopathy)
Hodgkin cycle
Hodgkin's
    disease
    granuloma
    paragranuloma
    sarcoma
Hofmann's bacillus
Hollenhorst plaques
holoacardius

Additional Entries

holoacardius *(continued)*
    h. acephalus
    h. acormus
    h. amorphus
Holophyra coli
Homalomyia
homocystinuria
homogentisuria
homonymous hemianopsia
homothallism
homozygous
    h. hemoglobinopathy
    h. thalassemia
    h.-type hemoglobin disorder
HOOD (hereditary osteo-onycho dysplasia)
hookworm
    American h.
    European h.
    New World h.
    Old World h.
Hormodendrum
    H. algeriensis
    H. carrionii
    H. compactum
    H. dermatitidis
    H. japonicum
    H. pedrosoi
    H. rossicum
Horner's syndrome
horror autotoxicus
horseshoe kidney
Horton's syndrome
Hottentot bustle
hottentotism
hourglass
    h. gallbladder

hourglass *(continued)*
    h. stomach
Houssay's syndrome
Howel-Evans' syndrome
Howship's lacuna
HPV (Hemophilus pertussis vaccine)
HS (hereditary spherocytosis, herpes simplex, Hurler's syndrome)
HSV (herpes simplex virus)
HSV I (herpes simplex virus I)
HSV II (herpes simplex virus II)
HT (Hypermetropia, total; hypertension)
Ht (total hyperopia)
HTHD (hypertensive heart disease)
HTLV (human T cell leukemia-lymphoma virus)
HTV (herpes-type virus)
HU (hydroxyurea)
Hua
    H. ningpoensis
    H. toucheana
Huchard's disease
Huet-Pelger nuclear anomaly
Huguenin's edema
human
    h. T cell leukemia-lymphoma virus
humpback (kyphosis)
Hunner's
    cystitis
    ulcer
Hunt's atrophy
Hunter's
    glossitis

Additional Entries

Hunter's *(continued)*
    syndrome
Huntington's chorea
Hurler's syndrome
Hurthle cell
    H. c. adenocarcinoma
    H. c. adenoma
    H. c. carcinoma
    H. c. metaplasia
HUS (hemolytic-uremic syndrome)
Hutchinson-Gilford syndrome
Hutchinson's
    disease
    melanotic freckle
Hutinel's disease
HV (herpesvirus)
HVD (hypertensive vascular disease)
HVH (herpesvirus hominis)
HVSD (hydrogen-detected ventricular septal defect)
Hy (hypermetropia)
hyalin
    alcoholic h.
hyaline
    h. arteriolosclerosis
    h. degeneration
    h. membrane disease
    h. perisplenitis
    h. thickening.
hyalinosis
    h. cutis et mucosae
hyalinuria
hyalitis
    h. punctata
    h. suppurativa
hyaloiditis (hyalitis)

Hyalomma
    H. aegyptium
hyaloserositis
    progressive multiple h.
hyalosis
    asteroid h.
hybridoma
hydatid
    alveolar h's
    h. degeneration
    h. mole
    Virchow's h.
hydatidiform mole
hydatidosis
hydatiduria
Hydatigera
    H. infantis
hydatism
hydradenitis (hidradenitis)
hydradenoma (hidradenoma)
hydramnios
hydranencephaly
hydrargyria
hydrargyromania
hydrargyrosis
hydrarthrodial
hydrarthrosis
    intermittent h.
hydremia
hydrencephalocele
hydrencephalomeningocele
hydrepigastrium
hydroa
    h. estivale
    h. vacciniforme
hydroadipsia
hydrocalycosis
hydrocele

Additional Entries

hydrocele *(continued)*
    cervical h.
    chylous h.
    h. coli
    communicating h.
    congenital h.
    diffused h.
    Dupuytren's h.
    encysted h.
    h. feminae
    funicular h.
    hernial h.
    Maunoir's h.
    h. of neck
    h. renalis
    h. sac
    scrotal h.
    h. spinalis
hydrocephalus
    communicating h.
    noncommunicating h.
    normal pressure h.
    normal pressure occult h.
    obstructive h.
    occult normal pressure h.
    otitic h.
    secondary h.
hydrocephaly
hydrocholecystis
hydrocholeresis
hydrocirsocele
hydrocolpos
hydrocyanism
hydrocyst
hydrocystadenoma
hydrocytosis
hydrodipsia
hydrodipsomania
hydrodiuresis
hydrohematonephrosis
hydrohepatosis
hydrohymenitis
hydromeningitis
hydromeningocele
hydrometra
hydrometrocolpos
hydromphalus
hydromyelia
hydromyelocele
hydromyelomeningocele
hydromyoma
hydronephrosis
    closed h.
    open h.
hydronephrotic
hydropancreatosis
hydroparotitis
hydropenia
hydropericarditis
hydroperinephrosis
hydroperitoneum
hydroperitonia
hydropexia
hydropexis
hydrophagocytosis
hydrophobia
    paralytic h.
hydrophthalmia
hydrophthalmos
    h. anterior
    h. posterior
    h. totalis
hydropneumatosis
hydropneumopericardium
hydropneumoperitoneum
hydropneumothorax

Additional Entries

hydrops
   h. abdominis
   h. ad matulam
   h. amnii
   h. articuli
   cochlear h.
   endolymphatic h.
   h. fetalis
   h. folliculi
   gallbladder h.
   labyrinthine h.
   h. percardii
   h. spurius
   h. tubae profluens
hydropyonephrosis
hydrorachis
hydrorachitis
hydrorrhea
   h. gravidarum
   nasal h.
hydrosalpinx
   h. follicularis
   intermittent h.
   h. simplex
hydrosarcocele
hydrosyringomyelia
Hydrotaea
   H. meteorica
hydrothorax
   chylous h.
hydrotympanum
hydroureter
hydroureteronephrosis
hydroxyprolinemia
hydroxyprolinuria
hydroxyurea
hygroma
   h. colli

hygroma *(continued)*
   cystic h.
   h. praepatellare
   subdural h.
Hylemyia
hymenitis
hymenolepiasis
Hymenolepididae
Hymenolepis
   H. diminuta
   H. lanceolata
   H. murina
   H. nana
Hymenomycetes
Hymenoptera
hypacidemia
hypalbuminemia
hypalgesia
hyperacidaminuria
hyperacidity
   gastric h.
hyperactivity
   motor h.
hyperacute
hyperadenosis
hyperadiposis
hyperadrenalism
hyperadrenocorticism
hyperalbuminemia
hyperalbuminosis
hyperaldosteronemia
hyperaldosteronism
hyperaldosteronuria
hyperalgesia
   auditory h.
   muscular h.
hyperalimentosis
hyperalkalinity

Additional Entries

hyperallantoinuria
hyperalonemia
hyperalphaglobulinemia
hyperalphalipoproteinemia
hyperaminoacidemia
hyperaminoaciduria
hyperammonemia
    cerebroatrophic h.
    congenital h., type I
    congenital h., type II
hyperammonuria
hyperamylasemia
hyperamylasuria
hyperargininemia
hyperarousal
hyperazotemia
hyperazoturia
hyper-beta-alaninemia
hyperbetaglobulinemia
hyperbetalipoproteinemia
    familial h.
hyperbicarbonatemia
hyperbilirubinemia
    congenital h.
    conjugated h.
    constitutional h.
    h. I
    neonatal h.
    unconjugated h.
hyperbilirubinuria
    obstructive h.
hyperblastosis
hyperbrachycephalic
hyperbradykinism
hypercalcemia
    familial hypocalciuric h.
    idiopathic h.
hypercalcipexy

hypercalcitoninemia
hypercalcitoninism
hypercalciuria
hypercapnia
hypercapnic
    h. acidosis
hypercarbia
hypercarotenemia
hypercatabolic
hypercatharsis
hypercellular
hypercementosis
hyperchloremia
hyperchloremic
hyperchlorhydria
hypercholesterinemia
hypercholesterolemia
    essential h.
    familial h.
hypercholia
hyperchondroplasia
hyperchromaffinism
hyperchromasia
hyperchromatism
hyperchromemia
hyperchromia
hyperchromic
hyperchylia
hyperchylomicronemia
    familial h.
hypercoagulability
hypercoagulable
hypercorticism
hypercorticosolism
hypercortisolism
hypercreatinemia
hypercryalgesia
hypercupremia

Additional Entries

hypercupriuria
hypercyanotic
hypercyesis
hypercythemia
hypercytosis
hyperdactyly
hyperdicrotic
hyperdipsia
hyperdistention
hyperdiuresis
hyperdontia
hyperdynamia
    h. uteri
hypereccrisia
hypereccritic
hyperechema
hyperechoic
hyperelastosis cutis
hyperelectrolytemia
hyperemesis
    h. gravidarum
    h. lactentium
hyperemetic
hyperemia
    active h.
    arterial h.
    collateral h.
    fluxionary h.
    leptomeningeal h.
    passive h.
    reactive h.
    venous h.
hyperencephalus
hypereosinophilia
    filarial h.
hyperepinephrinemia
hyperequilibrium
hyperergasia

hyperesophoria
hyperesthesia
    acoustic h.
    cerebral h.
    gustatory h.
    muscular h.
    olfactory h.
    oneiric h.
    optic h.
    tactile h.
hyperestrogenemia
hyperexcretory
hyperexophoria
hyperextension
hyperferremia
hyperfibrinogenemia
hyperflexion
hyperfunctioning
hypergalactia
hypergammaglobulinemia
    monoclonal h.
    polyclonal h.
hypergastrinemia
hyperglandular
hyperglobulinemia
hyperglycemia
hyperglycemic
    h. glycogenolytic factor
hyperglyceridemia
hyperglycinemia
    ketotic h.
    nonketotic h.
hyperglycinuria
hyperglycistia
hyperglycorrhachia
hyperglycosuria
hypergonadism
hypergonadotropic

Additional Entries

hyperhemoglobinemia
hyperheparinemia
hyperhepatia
hyperhidrosis
    h. unilateralis
hyperhidrotic
hyperhydration
hyperimmunoglobulinemia
    h. E
hyperinflation
hyperingestion
hyperinsulinemia
hyperiodemia
hyperirritability
hyperkalemia
hyperkaluria
hyperkeratosis
    h. eccentrica
    epidermolytic h.
    h. filiform
    follicular h.
    h. lacunaris
    h. lenticularis perstans
    h. of palms and soles
    h. penetrans
    progressive dystrophic h.
    h. subungualis
hyperkeratotic papilloma
hyperketonemia
hyperketonuria
hyperketosis
hyperkinesis
hyperlactacidemia
hyperlactation
hyperlecithinemia
hyperlethal
hyperleukocytosis
hyperleydigism

hyperlipemia
    carbohydrate-induced h.
    combined fat- and
        carbohydrate-induced h.
    familial h., essential
    fat-induced h., familial
    idiopathic h.
    mixed h.
hyperlipidemia
    carbohydrate-induced h.
    combined h., familial
    fat-induced h.
    multiple lipoprotein-type h.
hyperlipoproteinemia
    acquired h.
    broad-beta h., familial
    combined h., familial
    familial h.
    mixed h.
hyperliposis
hyperlordosis
hyperlucency
hyperluteinization
hyperlysinemia
hypermagnesemia
hypermastia
hypermelanosis
hypermenorrhea
hypermetabolic
hypermetabolism
    extrathyroidal h.
hypermetaplasia
hypermetria
hypermetropia
hypermobility
hypermyotonia

Additional Entries

hypermyotrophy
hypernatremia
    hypodipsic h.
hyperneocytosis
hypernephroma
hyperopia
    absolute h.
    axial h.
    curvature h.
    facultative h.
    index h.
    latent h.
    manifest h.
    relative h.
    total h.
hyperopic
hyperorchidism
hyperorexia
hyperorthocytosis
hyperosmia
hyperostosis
    h. corticalis deformans juvenilis
    h. corticalis generalisata
    h. cranii
    flowing h.
    h. frontalis interna
    infantile cortical h.
    Morgagni's h.
    senile ankylosing h. of spine
hyperovarianism
hyperoxaluria
    enteric h.
    primary h.
hyperoxemia
hyperoxia
hyperoxidation

hyperpallesthesia
hyperpancreorrhea
hyperparakeratosis
hyperparathyroidism
hyperpepsia
hyperpepsinemia
hyperpepsinuria
hyperperistalsis
    ureteral h.
hyperphagia
hyperphalangia
hyperphenylalaninemia
    malignant h.
hyperphosphatasemia
    chronic congenital idiopathic h.
    h. tarda
hyperphosphatasia
hyperphosphatemia
hyperphosphaturia
hyperpigmentation
hyperpinealism
hyperpituitarism
    postpubertal h.
    prepubertal h.
hyperplasia
    adenomatous h.
    adrenal cortical h.
    angiolymphoid h.
    atypical h.
    basal cell h.
    basophilic h.
    benign prostatic h.
    cementum h.
    chronic perforating pulp h.
    congenital adrenal h.
    congenital virilizing adrenal h.

Additional Entries

hyperplasia *(continued)*
    cutaneous lymphoid h.
    cystic endometrial h.
    diffuse h.
    endometrial h.
    eosinophilic h.
    erythroid h.
    fibrous inflammatory h.
    focal h.
    giant follicular h.
    gingival h.
    granulocytic h.
    hematopoietic h.
    inflammatory h.
    intracystic h.
    intraductal h.
    juxtaglomerular cell h.
    Leydig cell h.
    lipoid h.
    lipomelanotic reticuloendothelial cell h.
    lymphoid h.
    mast cell h.
    megakaryocytic h.
    myeloid h.
    neoplastic h.
    neutrophilic h.
    nodular lymphoid h.
    nodular mesothelial h.
    ovarian stromal h.
    papillary h.
    plasma cell h.
    polar h.
    polypoid h.
    primary h.
    pseudoepitheliomatous h.
    reserve cell h.

hyperplasia *(continued)*
    reticuloendothelial cell h.
    reticulum cell h.
    secondary h.
    stromal h.
    Swiss cheese h.
    wasserhelle h.
hyperplasmia
hyperplastic
    h. bone marrow
    h. nodular goiter
hyperpnea
hyperpneic
hyperpolarization
hyperpolypeptidemia
hyperponesis
hyperpotassemia
hyperprebetalipoproteinemia
hyperprolactinemia
hyperprolinemia
hyperproteinemia
hyperpyremia
hyperpyrexia
    malignant h.
hyperreactive
hyperreflexia
    autonomic h.
hyperreninemia
hypersalemia
hypersalivation
hypersarcosinemia
hypersecretion
    gastric h.
hypersegmentation
    hereditary h. of neutrophils
    leukocytic h.
hypersensitivity

Additional Entries

hypersensitivity *(continued)*
    contact h.
    cutaneous basophil h.
    delayed-type h.
    immediate h.
    tuberculin-type h.
hypersensitization
hyperserotonemia
hyperskeocytosis
hypersomatotropism
hypersomia
hypersomnia
hypersomnolence
hypersphyxia
hypersplenia
hypersplenism
hypersplenosis
hyperspongiosis
hypersteatosis
hypersthenia
hypersthenuria
hypersympathicotonus
hypertarachia
hypertelorism
    ocular h., orbital h.
hypertension
    accelerated h.
    adrenal h.
    benign intracranial h.
    borderline h.
    diastolic h.
    essential h.
    Goldblatt's h.
    idiopathic h.
    intracranial h.
    labile h.
    low-renin h.
    malignant h.

hypertension *(continued)*
    mineralocorticoid h.
    neuromuscular h.
    ocular h.
    orthostatic h.
    pale h.
    paroxysmal h.
    portal h.
    primary h.
    pulmonary h.
    red h.
    renal h.
    renovascular h.
    secondary h.
    splenoportal h.
    symptomatic h.
    systemic venous h.
    systolic h.
    vascular h.
hypertensive
    h. cardiovascular disease
    h. heart disease
hyperthecosis
hyperthelia
hyperthermalgesia
hyperthermesthesia
hyperthermia
    malignant h.
hyperthrombinemia
hyperthymia
hyperthyroidism
    masked h.
hyperthyroiditis
hyperthyroxinemia
    familial dysalbuminemic h.
hypertonia
    h. polycythaemica

Additional Entries

hypertonicity
hypertonus
hypertoxic
hypertrichosis
    h. lanuginosa
    h. pinnae auris
    h. universalis
hypertriglyceridemia
    carbohydrate-induced h.
    familial h.
hypertrophia
hypertrophic
    h. amphophil cell
    h. arthritis
    h. chronic vulvitis
    h. fibrous pachymeningitis
    h. gastritis
    h. lichen planus
    h. osteoarthropathy
    h. polyneuritic-type muscular atrophy
    h. pulmonary osteoarthropathy
    h. pyloric stenosis
hypertrophy
    adaptive h.
    benign prostatic h.
    Billroth h.
    compensatory h.
    complementary h.
    concentric h.
    diffuse h.
    eccentric h.
    false h.
    fibrocongestive h.
    focal h.
    functional h.
    giant rugal h.

hypertrophy *(continued)*
    hemifacial h.
    Marie's h.
    numeric h.
    physiologic h.
    pseudomuscular h.
    quantitative h.
    simple h.
    true h.
    unilateral h.
    ventricular h.
    vicarious h.
hypertropia
hypertyrosinemia
hyperuremia
hyperuricemia
hyperuricosuria
hyperuricuria
hyperurobilinogenemia
hypervalinemia
hyperventilation
hyperviscosity
hypervitaminosis
    h. A
    h. D
hypervolemia
hypesthesia
    tactile h.
    thermal h.
hyphema
Hyphomyces destruens
hyphomycosis
hypnagogic
    h. hypersynchrony
hypoacidity
hypoactive
hypoadrenalism
hypoadrenocorticism

Additional Entries

hypoalbuminemia
hypoalbuminosis
hypoaldosteronism
hypoalkalinity
hypoalphaglobulinemia
hypobaropathy
hypobetalipoproteinemia
    familial h.
hypobilirubinemia
hypocalcemia
hypocalciuria
hypocapnia
hypocarbia
hypochloremia
hypochlorhydria
hypocholesterolemia
hypocholuria
hypochondriasis
hypochondroplasia
hypochromasia
hypochromatism
hypochromemia
    idiopathic h.
hypochromia
hypochromic
    h. anemia
    h. microcytic anemia
hypochromotrichia
hypochrosis
hypochylia
hypocomplementemia
hypocupremia
hypocyclosis
hypocythemia
hypocytosis
hypodactyly
Hypoderma
    H. bovis

Hypoderma *(continued)*
    H. lineatum
hypodermiasis
hypodermolithisis
hypodiploid
hypodipsia
hypodontia
hypodynamia
    h. cordis
hypoeccrisia
hypoeccrisis
hypoelectrolytemia
hypoeosinophilia
hypoepinephrinemia
hypoequilibrium
hypoergasia
hypoesophoria
hypoesthesia
    acoustic h.
    gustatory h.
    olfactory h.
    tactile h.
hypoestrogenemia
hypoevolution
hypoexophoria
hypoferremia
hypofertile
hypofibrinogenemia
hypogalactia
hypogammaglobulinemia
    acquired h.
    common variable h.
    congenital h.
    physiologic h.
    transient h. of infancy
    Swiss-type h.
    X-linked h., X-linked
        infantile h.

Additional Entries

hypoganglionosis
hypogastroschisis
hypogenesis
    polar h.
hypogeusia
hypoglandular
hypoglobulinemia
hypoglucagonemia
hypoglycemia
    factitial h.
    fasting h.
    ketotic h.
    leucine-induced h.
    mixed h.
    reactive h.
hypoglycemosis
hypoglycorrhachia
hypognathus
hypogonadism
    eugonadotropic h.
    hypergonadotropic h.
    hypogonadotropic h.
    primary h.
    secondary h.
hypogonadotropic
hypogranulocytosis
hypohepatia
hypohidrosis
hypohidrotic
hypohydration
hypoinsulinemia
hypoinsulinism
hypoiodidism
hypokalemia
hypokalemic
    h. nephropathy
    h. nephrosis
hypokaluria

hypolactasia
hypoleydigism
hypolipoproteinemia
hypolymphemia
hypomagnesemia
hypomania
hypomanic
    h. personality
    h.-type manic-depressive
        psychosis
hypomastia
hypomelancholia
hypomelanosis
    idiopathic guttate h.
    h. of Ito
hypomenorrhea
hypometabolic
hypometabolism
hypometria
hypomineralization
hypomotility
hypomyotonia
hypomyxia
hyponatremia
    depletional h.
    dilutional h.
    hyperlipemic h.
hyponatruria
hyponeocytosis
hyponitremia
hyponoia
hyponychon
hypo-orchidism
hypo-orthocytosis
hypo-ovarianism
hypopancreatism
hypopancreorrhea
hypoparathyroidism

Additional Entries

hypopepsia
hypopepsinia
hypoperfusion
hypoperistalsis
hypopexia
hypophalangism
hypophoria
hypophosphatasia
hypophosphatemia
    X-linked familial h.
hypophosphaturia
hypophrenia
hypophysitis
hypopiesia
hypopiesis
hypopietic
hypopigmentation
hypopituitarism
hypoplasia
    cartilage-hair h.
    enamel h.
    erythroid h.
    focal dermal h.
    granulocytic h.
    hematopoietic h.
    lymphoid h.
    megakaryocytic h.
    oligomeganephronic renal h.
    h. of right ventricle
    thymic h.
    Turner's h.
hypoplastic
    h. anemia
    h. bone marrow
hypoploid
hypopnea
hypopneic

hypoponesis
hypoporosis
hypoposia
hypopotassemia
hypopotentia
hypopraxia
hypoproaccelerinemia
hypoproconvertinemia
hypoproteinemia
    prehepatic h.
hypoprothrombinemia
hypoptyalism
hypopyon
hyporeactive
hyporeflexia
hyporeninemia
hyporeninemic
hyporrhea
hyposalemia
hyposalivation
hyposecretion
hyposensitization
hyposmia
hyposomatotropism
hyposomia
hyposomnia
hypospadiac
hypospadias
    balanic h., balanitic h.
    female h.
    glandular h.
    penile h.
    penoscrotal h.
    perineal h.
    pseudovaginal h.
hyposplenism
hypostasis
hypostatic pneumonia

Additional Entries

hyposteatolysis
hyposthenia
hyposthenuria
    tubular h.
hypostomia
hypostosis
hyposympathicotonus
hyposynergia
hyposystole
hypotelorism
    ocular h.
hypotension
hypothermia
    endogenous h.
    orthostatic h.
    postural h.
    vascular h.
hypothrepsia
hypothrombinemia
hypothymia
hypothyroid
hypothyroidism
hypotonia
    benign congenital h.
    h. oculi
    vasomotor h.
hypotonic
hypotonicity
hypotonus
hypotransferrinemia
hypotrichiasis
hypotrichosis
hypotropia
hypotryptophanic
hypouremia
hypouricemia
hypouricuria
hypourocrinia

hypovenosity
hypoventilation
hypovitaminosis
hypovolemia
hypovolemic
hypoxemia
hypoxia
    anemic h.
    histotoxic h.
    hypoxic h.
    ischemic h.
    stagnant h.
hypoxic
hypoxidosis
hypsarrhythmia
hypsokinesis
hypsonosus
hysteralgia
hysteratresia
hysteria
    anxiety h.
    canine h.
    conversion h.
    dissociative h.
    fixation h.
    h. major
hysterical
hysterobubonocele
hysterocarcinoma
hysterocele
hysterodynia
hysteroepilepsy
hysterolith
hysteromyoma
hysteropathy
hysteroptosia
hysteroptosis
hysterorrhexis
hysterovaginoenterocele

Additional Entries

I

IADHS (inappropriate antidiuretic hormone syndrome)
IASD (interatrial septal defect)
iatrogenic anemia
IC (intermittent claudication; irritable colon)
ICA (intracranial aneurysm)
ICAO (internal carotid artery occlusion)
ICC (Indian childhood cirrhosis)
ichorrhea
ichorrhemia
ichthyoacanthotoxism
ichthyohemotoxism
ichthyosarcotoxism
ichthyosis
    i. congenita
    i. hystrix
    lamellar i.
    i. linearis circumflexa
    i. linguae
    i. palmaris et plantaris
    i. simplex
    i. uteri
    i. vulgaris
    X-linked i.
ICT (inflammation of connective tissue; insulin coma therapy)
ictal
icteric
icteroanemia
icterogenic
    i. spirochetosis
icterohematuria
icterohematuric
icterohemoglobinuria
icterohepatitis
icteroid
Icterohemorrhagiae
    I. leptospirosis
icterus
    chronic familial i.
    congenital familial i.
    epidemic catarrhal i.
    i. gravis
    i. gravis neonatorum
    i. interference
    i. neonatorum
    nuclear i.
    i. praecox
    i. typhoides
ictus
    i. cordis
    i. epilepticus
    i. paralyticus
    i. sanguinis
    i. solis
IDA (iron deficiency anemia)
IDDM (insulin-dependent diabetes mellitus)
idiocy
    amaurotic familial i.
    athetosic i.
    Aztec i.
    cretinoid i.
    juvenile amaurotic familial i.
    Kalmuk i.
    microcephalic i.

Additional Entries

idiocy *(continued)*
    mongolian i.
    spastic amaurotic axonal i.
    xerodermic i.
idiopathic
    i. etiology
    i. generalized
        glycogenesis
    i. hemosiderosis
    i. hypertrophic subaortic
        stenosis
idiopathy
    toxic i.
idiosyncrasy
idiosyncratic
idiot
    mongolian i.
    i.-savant
idiotoxin
idioventricular rhythm
IDS (immunity deficiency state)
IgA (immunodeficiency
    nephropathy)
IH (infectious hepatitis)
IHBTD (incompatible hemolytic
    blood transfusion disease)
IHC (idiopathic hypercalciuria)
IHD (ischemic heart disease)
IHO (idiopathic hypertrophic
    osteoarthropathy)
IHSS (idiopathic hypertrophic
    subaortic stenosis)
ILD (ischemic leg disease;
    ischemic limb disease)
ileitis
    distal i.
    regional i.
    terminal i.

ileocolitis
    tuberculous i.
    i. ulcerosa chronica
ileus
    adynamic i.
    dynamic i.
    gallstone i.
    mechanical i.
    meconium i.
    occlusive i.
    paralytic i.
    spastic i.
    i. subparta
    ureteral i.
Ilheus virus
illness
    compressed-air i.
    high-altitude i.
    manic-depressive i.
    mental i.
    psychosomatic i.
    radiation i.
IM (infectious mononucleosis)
IMB (intermenstrual bleeding)
imbalance
    autonomic i.
    binocular i.
    electrolyte i.
    sympathetic i.
    vasomotor i.
imbecile
imbecility
    moral i.
    phenylpyruvic i.
IMH (idiopathic myocardial
    hypertrophy)
iminoglycinuria
immersion syndrome

Additional Entries

immotile cilia syndrome
immune
    i. complex diseases
    i. complex
        glomerulopathy
    i. complex nephropathy
immunodeficiency
    combined i.
    common variable i.
    i. with hyper-IgM
    severe combined i. (SCID)
    i. with short-limbed
        dwarfism
    i. with thymoma
immunodepression
immunodeviation
immunoglobulinopathy
immunoincompetent
immunologic
    i. paralysis
    i. unresponsiveness
immunoparalysis
immunopathogenesis
immunopathology
immunoproliferative
    i. small intestinal disease
immunosuppression
impacted
    i. feces
    i. fracture
    i. tooth
impaction
    ceruminal i.
    dental i.
    fecal i.
    food i.
impalpable
imperforate

imperforation
impetigo
    Bockhart's i.
    i. bullosa
    i. contagiosa
    i. herpetiformis
    staphylococcal i.
    streptococcal i.
    i. vulgaris
impotence
    sexual i.
impotentia
    i. coeundi
    i. erigendi
    i. generandi
IMR (infant mortality rate)
INAD (infantile neuroaxonal
  dystrophy)
in articulo mortis
inborn
    i. error of metabolism
incarcerated hernia
inclusion
    i. blenorrhea
    i. conjunctivitis
    i. conjunctivitis virus
    i. cyst, epidermal
    i. cyst, epidermoid
    i. cyst, epithelial
    i. cyst, germinal
    i. cyst, germinal epithelial
    cytoplasmic i.
incompatibility
    ABO i.
    chemical i.
    physiologic i.
incompetence
    valvular i.

Additional Entries

incompetency and stenosis,
  mitral
incompetent
  i. aortic valve
  i. foramen ovale valve
  i. mitral valve
  i. pulmonic valve
  i. tricuspid valve
incomplete
  i. abortion
  i. amnion
  i. amputation
  i. compound fracture
  i. conjoined twins
  i. differentiation, cardiac
    valve
  i. dislocation
  i. hernia
  i. regeneration
incontinence
  active i.
  fecal i.
  intermittent i.
  over-flow i.
  paradoxical i.
  paralytic i.
  passive i.
  rectal i.
  stress i.
  urinary i.
incontinentia
  Naegeli's i. pigmenti
  i. pigmenti
  i. pigmenti achromians
  i. urinae
incyclotropia
Indian rat flea
indigenous

indigenous *(continued)*
  i. bacterium
indigestion
  acid i.
  fat i.
  gastric i.
  intestinal i.
  nervous i.
  sugar i.
indirect hernia
indoleaceturia
indoluria
indoxyluria
induced
  i. abortion
  i. allergic
    encephalomyelitis
  i. allergic neuritis
  i. glomerulonephritis
  i. thyroiditis
  i. uveitis
induration
  black i.
  brawny i.
  brown i.
  cyanotic i.
  fibroid i.
  Froriep's i.
  granular i.
  gray i.
  laminate i.
  parchment i.
  penile i.
  phlebitic i.
  plastic i.
  red i.
INE (infantile necrotizing
  encephalomyelopathy)

Additional Entries

Inermicapsifer
    I. madagascariensis
inertia
    colonic i.
    immunological i.
    i. uteri
in extremis
infantile
    i. amaurotic familial idiocy
    i. hemangioma
    i. muscular atrophy
    i. progressive spinal muscular dystrophy
    i. respiratory distress syndrome
    i. spasm
    i. type coarctation
    i. uterus
infantilism
    Brissaud's i.
    cachetic i.
    celiac i.
    dysthyroidal i.
    hepatic i.
    Herter's i.
    hypophysial i.
    intestinal i.
    Levi-Lorain i.
    lymphatic i.
    myxedematous i.
    pancreatic i.
    partial i.
    pituitary i.
    regressive i.
    renal i.
    sexual i.
    symptomatic i.

infantilism *(continued)*
    universal i.
infarct
    acute i.
    anemic i.
    bilirubin i's
    bland i.
    bone i.
    Brewer's i.
    calcareous i.
    cerebral i.
    cystic i.
    embolic i.
    focal i.
    healed i.
    hemorrhagic i.
    microscopic i.
    old i.
    pale i.
    pulmonary i.
    recent i.
    red i.
    ruptured myocardial i.
    septic i.
    thrombotic i.
    uric acid i.
    white i.
    Zahn's i.
infarction
    anterior myocardial i.
    anteroinferior myocardial i.
    anterolateral myocardial i.
    anteroseptal myocardial i.
    atrial i.
    cardiac i.
    cerebral i.
    Freiberg's i.

Additional Entries

infarction *(continued)*
    inferior myocardial i.
    inferolateral myocardial i.
    intestinal i.
    lateral myocardial i.
    mesenteric i.
    myocardial i.
    posterior myocardial i.
    pulmonary i.
    renal i.
    septal myocardial i.
    transmural myocardial i.
infect
infection
    airborne i.
    apical i.
    colonization i.
    cryptogenic i.
    droplet i.
    dust-borne i.
    ectogenous i.
    endogenous i.
    exogenous i.
    germinal i.
    iatrogenic i.
    inapparent i.
    latent i.
    mass i.
    mixed i.
    nosocomial i.
    opportunistic i.
    pyogenic i.
    Salinem i.
    secondary i.
    subclinical i.
    vector-borne i.
    Vincent's i.
    water-borne i.
infectious
    i. agent
    i. arteritis
    i. disease
    i. hepatitis
    i. mononucleosis
    i. parotitis
    i. wastes
infertility
    primary i.
    secondary i.
infestation
infiltrate
    acute inflammatory i.
    Assmann's tuberculous i.
    eosinophil leukocytic i.
    inflammatory i.
    leukocytic i.
    lymphocytic inflammatory i.
    monocytic inflammatory i.
    neutrophilic i.
    plasma cell i.
    polymorphonuclear leukocytic i.
infiltrating
    i. comedocarcinoma
    i. duct adenocarcinoma
    i. duct carcinoma
    i. lobular carcinoma
infiltration
    adipose i.
    calcareous i.
    calcium i.
    cellular i.
    epituberculous i.
    fatty i.
    gelatinous i.

Additional Entries

infiltration *(continued)*
    glycogen i.
    gray i.
    inflammatory i.
    lymphocytic i. of skin
    paraneural i.
    sanguineous i.
    serous i.
    tuberculous i.
    urinous i.
infiltrative fasciitis
inflammation
    active chronic i.
    acute i.
    acute and chronic i.
    adhesive i.
    atrophic i.
    blenorrhagic i.
    bullous i.
    bullous granulomatous i.
    calcified granulomatous i.
    caseating i.
    caseous i.
    catarrhal i.
    chronic i.
    circumscribed i.
    cirrhotic i.
    confluent i.
    croupous i.
    cystic i.
    cystic granulomatous i.
    diffuse i.
    disseminated i.
    erosive i.
    exanthematous i.
    exudative i.
    exudative granulomatous i.

inflammation *(continued)*
    fibrinoid necrotizing i.
    fibrinopurulent i.
    fibrinous i.
    fibrocaseous i.
    fibroid i.
    focal granulomatous i.
    follicular i.
    gangrenous i.
    gangrenous granulomatous i.
    gelatinous i.
    granulomatous i.
    gummatous i.
    hemorrhagic i.
    hyperplastic i.
    hypertrophic i.
    interstitial i.
    localized i.
    membranous i.
    metastatic i.
    miliary granulomatous i.
    multifocal i.
    necrotizing i.
    necrotizing granulomatous i.
    non-necrotizing granulomatous i.
    obliterative i.
    organizing i.
    ossifying i.
    parenchymatous i.
    plastic i.
    proliferative i.
    pseudomembranous i.
    purulent i.
    pustular i.
    recurrent i.

Additional Entries

inflammation *(continued)*
- sclerosing i.
- seroplastic i.
- serous i.
- simple i.
- subacute i.
- subsiding i.
- suppurative i.
- suppurative granulomatous i.
- toxic i.
- transudative i.
- traumatic i.
- ulcerative i.
- uremic i.
- vesicular i.
- vesicular granulomatous i.

inflammatory
- i. adenocarcinoma
- i. bowel disease
- i. carcinoma
- i. cavity
- i. cyst
- i. exudate
- i. fistula
- i. infiltrate
- i. infiltrate, lymphocytic
- i. infiltrate, monocytic
- i. membrane
- i. necrosis
- i. perforation
- i. polyp
- i. pseudomembrane
- i. pseudotumor
- i. reaction
- i. rupture
- i. sinus
- i. sinus tract

inflammatory *(continued)*
- i. transudate

influenza
- i. A
- Asian i.
- avian i.
- i. B
- i. C
- endemic i.
- equine i.
- feline i.
- goose i.
- Hong Kong i.
- laryngeal i.
- Russian i.
- Spanish i.
- swine i.

infundiboloma
inguinal hernia
inhalation pneumonia
iniencephaly
initis
inochondritis
inohymenitis
inomyositis
inositis
insomnia
insufficiency
- active i.
- adrenal i.
- aortic i.
- cardiac i.
- circulatory i.
- coronary i.
- i. of the externi
- i. of the eyelids
- gastric i.
- gastromotor i.

Additional Entries

insufficiency *(continued)*
    hepatic i.
    ileocecal i.
    i. of the interni
    mitral i.
    muscular i.
    myocardial i.
    parathyroid i.
    placental i.
    pulmonary i.
    renal i.
    respiratory i.
    thyroid i.
    tricuspid i.
    uterine i.
    i. of the valves
    velopharyngeal i.
    venous i.
    vertebrobasilar i.
insulinoma
insulitis
interatrial septal defect
interchromosomal aberration
intermittent claudication
interstitial
    i. cell tumor
    i. emphysema
    i. fibrosis
    i. inflammation
    i. nephritis
    i. nephropathy
    i. pneumonia
intestinal
    i. flow disorder
    i. fluke
    i. lipodystrophy
    i. lymphangiectasia
    i. metaplasia

intestinal *(continued)*
    i. myiasis
    i. obstruction
intolerance
    disaccharide i.
    drug i.
    hereditary fructose i.
    lactose i.
    lactose i., congenital
    lysine i., congenital
    lysinuric protein i.
    sucrose i., congenital
intoxication
    acid i.
    alcohol idiosyncratic i.
    alkaline i.
    bongkrek i.
    intestinal i.
    pathological i.
    roentgen i.
    serum i.
    vitamin D i.
    water i.
intrachromosomal aberration
intracystic
    i. hyperplasia
    i. papilloma
intradermal nevus
intraductal
    i. carcinoma
    i. hyperplasia
    i. papilloma
    i. papillomatosis
intraepidermal
    i. basal cell epithelioma, Borst-Jadassohn
    i. carcinoma
    i. nevus

Additional Entries

intumescentia
    i. cervicalis
    i. lumbalis
    i. lumbosacralis
    i. tympanica
intussusception
    agonic i., postmortem i.
    retrograde i.
inverted
    i. follicular keratosis
    i. keratosis
IO (intestinal obstruction)
Iodamoeba
    I. butschlii
    I. williamsi
iododerma
IPD (inflammatory pelvic disease)
IPH (idiopathic pulmonary hemosiderosis)
IPSID (immunoproliferative small intestinal disease)
IRBBB (incomplete right bundle branch block)
IRDS (idiopathic respiratory distress syndrome; infant respiratory distress syndrome)
iridalgia
iridauxesis
iridemia
irideremia
iridocapsulitis
iridocele
iridochoroiditis
iridocoloboma
iridocyclitis
    heterochromic i.

iridocyclochoroiditis
iridodiastasis
iridodonesis
iridokeratitis
iridoleptynsis
iridomalacia
iridopathy
iridoperiphakitis
iridoplegia
    accommodation i.
    complete i.
    reflex i.
    sympathetic i.
iridoptosis
iridorhexis
iridoschisis
iridosteresis
iridovirus
irisopsia
iritis
    i. catamenialis
    diabetic i.
    follicular i.
    gouty i.
    i. papulosa
    plastic i.
    purulent i.
    serous i.
    spongy i.
    sympathetic i.
    uratic i.
iron
    i. deficiency anemia
    i. storage disease
irovirus
irregular pulse
irreversibly sickled cell
irritability

Additional Entries

irritability *(continued)*
    i. of the bladder
    nervous i.
    i. of the stomach
irritable bowel syndrome
Isambert's disease
ISC (irreversibly sickled cell)
ischemia
    myocardial i.
    i. retinae
ischemic
    i. cardiomyopathy
    i. heart disease
    i. necrosis
ISH (icteric serum hepatitis)
islet cell
    i. c. adenoma
    i. c. carcinoma
    i. c. hyperinsulinism
    i. c. hyperplasia
isoimmune hemolytic anemia
isoimmunization
    Rh i. syndrome
Isoparorchis
    I. hypselobagri
    I. trisimilitubis
Isospora
    I. belli
    I. hominis
isosporiasis
isovalericacidemia
Itaqui virus
itch
    Aujeszky's i.
    baker's i.
    barber's i.
    clam diggers' i.
    copra i.

itch *(continued)*
    Cuban i.
    dew i.
    dhobie mark i.
    grain i.
    grocers' i.
    ground i.
    jock i.
    mad i.
    prairie i.
    seven-year i.
    straw i.
    swimmer's i.
    winter i.
ithylordosis
ithyokyphosis
ITP (idiopathic thrombocytopenic purpura)
IUM (intrauterine fetally malnourished)
IVH (intraventricular hemorrhage)
IVM (intravascular mass)
IVSD (interventricular septal defect)
Iwanoff's cysts
Ixodes
    I. bicornis
    I. cavipalpus
    I. frequens
    I. holocyclus
    I. pacificus
    I. persulcatus
    I. rasus
    I. ricinus
    I. scapularis
ixodiasis
ixodic

Additional Entries

Ixodides
Ixodiphagus

Ixodiphagus *(continued)*
    I. caucurtei
Ixodoidea

Additional Entries

J

Jaccoud's fever
Jackson's sign
jacksonian
    j. epilepsy
    j. motor seizure
Jacob's ulcer
Jacobson's retinitis
Jacquet's dermatitis
Jadassohn's
    anetoderma
    sebaceous nevus
Jadassohn's nevus
Jadassohn-Pellizari anetoderma
Jakob's disease
Jakob-Creutzfeldt
    disease
    pseudosclerosis
Jaksch's disease
Janet's disease
Janeway's lesion
Jansen's disease
Japanese B encephalitis virus
jaundice
    acholuric j.
    acholuric familial j.
    anhepatic j.
    black j.
    breast milk j.
    cholestatic j.
    congenital familial
        nonhemolytic j.
    Criger-Najjar j.
    epidemic j.
    familial nonhemolytic j.
    hemolytic h.

jaundice *(continued)*
    hepatocellular j.
    infectious j.
    Israels' familial j.
    latent j.
    leptospiral j.
    malignant j.
    mechanical j.
    j. of the newborn
    nonhemolytic j.
    nuclear j.
    obstructive j.
    physiologic j.
    picric acid j.
    post-arsphenamine j.
    regurgitation j.
    retention j.
    Schmori's j.
    spirochetal j.
    toxemic j.
Jeanselme's nodules
JBE (Japanese B encephalitis)
jejunitis
jejunoileitis
Jellinek's sign
Jensen's sarcoma
jet lesion
JH virus
Job's syndrome
jock itch
Jod-Basedow phenomenon
Johne's bacillus
Johnson-Stevens disease
Joseph's disease

Additional Entries

JRA (juvenile rheumatoid arthritis)
Junin virus
juvenile
    j. angiofibroma
    j. diabetes mellitus
    j. fibroadenoma

juvenile *(continued)*
    j. melanoma
    j. pernicious anemia
    j. pilocytic astrocytoma
    j. polyposis
    j. rheumatoid arthritis
    j. xanthogranuloma
    j. xanthoma

Additional Entries

K

KA (ketoacidosis)
Kahler's disease
kaliopenia
Kallmann's syndrome
Kalmuk idiocy
Kanavel's sign
Kanner's syndrome
kanyemba
kaolinosis
Kaposi's
    sarcoma
    varicelliform eruption
Karroo syndrome
Kartagener's syndrome
karyopyknosis
karyorrhectic
karyorrhexis
Kasabach-Merritt syndrome
Kawasaki disease
Kayser's disease
Kearns-Sayre syndrome
Kennedy's syndrome
Kerandel's sign
keraphyllocele
keratansulfaturia
keratectasia
keratinization
    metaplastic k.
keratitis
    acne rosacea k.
    actinic k.
    aerosol k.
    alphabet k.
    anaphylactic k.
    annular k.

keratitis *(continued)*
    k. arborescens
    artificial silk k.
    aspergillus k.
    band-shaped k.
    k. bullosa
    catarrhal ulcerative k.
    deep k.
    deep pustular k.
    dendriform k.
    desiccation k.
    Dimmer's k.
    k. disciformis
    epithelial diffuse k.
    exfoliative k.
    exposure k.
    fascicular k.
    k. filamentosa
    furrow k.
    herpetic k.
    interstitial k.
    lagophthalmic k.
    lattice k.
    marginal k.
    metaherpetic k.
    mycotic k.
    neuroparalytic k.
    neurotrophic k.
    k. nummularis
    parenchymatous k.
    k. petrificans
    phlyctenular k.
    k. profunda
    k. punctata leprosa
    k. punctata profunda

Additional Entries

keratitis *(continued)*
    k. punctata subepithelialis
    punctate k., deep
    punctate k., superficial
    purulent k.
    k. pustuliformis profunda
    reaper's k.
    reticular k.
    ribbon-like k.
    rosacea k.
    sclerosing k.
    secondary k.
    serpiginous k.
    striate k.
    suppurative k.
    trachomatous k.
    trophic k.
    vascular k.
    vesicular k.
    xerotic k.
    zonular k.
keratoacanthoma
keratocele
keratoconjunctivitis
    epidemic k.
    flash k.
    phlyctenular k.
    shipyard k.
    k. sicca
    viral k.
keratoconus
keratoderma
    k. acquisitum
    k. blennorrhagicum
    k. climactericum
    k. palmare et plantare
    palmoplantar k., diffuse
keratodermatocele

keratohelcosis
keratohemia
keratoiditis
keratoiridocyclitis
keratoiritis
    hypopyon k.
keratoleukoma
keratolysis
    pitted k., k. plantare sulcatum
keratoma
    k. hereditarium mutilans
    k. plantare sulcatum
    k. senile
keratomalacia
keratomycosis
    k. linguae
keratonosus
keratopathy
    band k.
    bullous k.
    climatic k.
    filamentary k.
    Labrador k.
    lipid k.
    striate k.
    vesicular k.
keratophakia
keratorhexis
keratoscleritis
keratosis
    actinic k.
    arsenical k.
    k. blennorrhagica
    k. follicularis
    k. follicularis contagiosa
    inverted k.
    inverted follicular k.

Additional Entries

keratosis *(continued)*
    k. linguae
    k. obturans
    pilaris k.
    k. palmaris et plantaris
    k. pharyngea
    seborrheic k.
    senile k.
    solar k.
    stucco k.
    tar k.
keratotic
    k. papilloma
    k. precipitates
keratotorus
kerectasis
kernicterus
Kernig's sign
Keshan disease
ketoacidemia
    branched-chain k.
ketoacidosis
ketoaciduria
    branched-chain k.
ketoaminoacidemia
ketonemia
ketonuria
ketosis
ketosuria
KFS (Klippel-Feil syndrome)
kidney
    abdominal k.
    Armanni-Ebstein k.
    arteriosclerotic k.
    atrophic k.
    cake k.
    cicatricial k.
    congested k.

kidney *(continued)*
    contracted k.
    cystic k.
    disk k.
    doughnut k.
    fatty k.
    flea-bitten k.
    floating k.
    Formad's k.
    fused k.
    Goldblatt's k.
    horseshoe k.
    lardaceous k.
    lumbar k.
    lump k.
    medullary sponge k.
    myelin k.
    myeloma k.
    mural k.
    polycystic k.
    putty k.
    Rokitansky's k.
    Rose-Bradford k.
    sacciform k.
    sigmoid k.
    sponge k.
    thoracic k.
    wandering k.
    waxy k.
Kienbock's disease
Kimmelstiel-Wilson
    lesion
    syndrome
Kimura's disease
kinesalgia
kinesioneurosis
Kingella
    K. denitrificans

Additional Entries

Kingella *(continued)*
    K. indologenes
    K. kingae
Kirchner's diverticulum
Klebsiella
    K. friedlanderi
    K. oxytoca
    K. ozaenae
    K. pneumoniae
    K. rhinoscleromatis
    K. terrigena
Klebsielleae
Klebs-Loffler bacillus
kleeblattschadel
Kleine-Levin syndrome
Klinefelter's syndrome
Klippel's disease
Klippel-Trenaunay syndrome
Klumpke's paralysis
Klumpke-Dejerine
    paralysis
    syndrome
Kluver-Bucy syndrome
Kluyvera
Koch's bacillus
Koch-Weeks
    bacillus
    hemophilus
Kogoj's abscess
Kohler's disease
koilocytotic atypia
koilonychia
Konig's syndrome
Koplik's spots
Kopp's asthma
Koranyi's sign

Korsakoff's syndrome
Koshevnikoff's disease
Kostmann's syndrome
Krabbe's
    disease
    leukodystrophy
kraurosis
    k. vulvae
Kreysig's sign
Krishaber's disease
Krompecher's carcinoma
Krukenberg's tumor
KS (Klinefelter's syndrome)
kubisagari
Kufs' disease
Kumba virus
Kummell's disease
Kummell-Verneuil disease
Kunkel's syndrome
Kupffer's cell sarcoma
kurtosis
Kussmaul's aphasia
Kussmaul-Kien respiration
Kussmaul-Landry paralysis
Kussmaul-Maier disease
kwashiorkor
    marasmic k.
Kyasanur Forest
    disease
    disease virus
kyllosis
kyphoscoliosis
kyphosis
    k. dorsalis juvenilis;
        Scheuermann's k.
Kyrle's disease

Additional Entries

L

L. (Lactobacillus)
labiomycosis
lactacidemia
Lactarius
    L. torminosus
lactating adenoma
lactic
    l. acid bacteria
    l. acidosis
Lactobacillaceae
Lactobacillus
    L. acidophilus
    L. arabinosus
    L. bifidus
    L. brevis
    L. bulgaricus
    L. casei
    L. catenaforme
    L. cellobiosus
    L. fermentans
    L. fermenti
    L. jensenii
    L. leichmannii
    L. plantarum
lactobacillus
    l. of Boas-Oppler
Lactobacteriaceae
lactosidosis
lactosuria
lactosyl ceramidosis
LAE (left atrial enlargement)
Laennec's
    catarrh
    cirrhosis
Lafora's disease
Lagochilascaris minor
lagophthalmos
LAH (left atrial hypertrophy)
lalopathy
laloplegia
Lamblia (Giardia)
    L. intestinalis (Giardia lamblia)
lambliasis, lambliosis
lamellar necrosis
laminitis
Lancereaux-Mathieu disease
Landouzy's disease
Landouzy-Dejerine progressive muscular dystrophy
Landry's paralysis
Langdon Down's disease (Down's syndrome)
Lansing virus
laparocele
laparomonodidymus
laparomyitis
Larsen's disease
Larsen-Johansson disease
laryngalgia
laryngismus
    l. paralyticus
    l. stridulus
laryngitis
    acute catarrhal l.
    atrophic l.
    chronic catarrhal l.
    croupous l.
    diphtheritic l.
    membranous l.
    necrotic l.

Additional Entries

laryngitis *(continued)*
   phlegmonous l.
   l. sicca
   l. stridulosa
   subglottic l.
   syphilitic l.
   tuberculous l.
   vestibular l.
laryngocele
   ventricular l.
laryngomalacia
laryngoparalysis
laryngopathy
laryngopharyngitis
laryngophthsis
laryngoplegia
laryngoptosis
laryngopyocele
laryngorrhagia
laryngorrhea
laryngoscleroma
laryngospasm
laryngostasis
laryngostenosis
laryngotracheitis
laryngotracheobronchitis
laryngovestibulitis
laryngoxerosis
Lasegue's sign
Lassa virus
lathyrism
Latrodectus
   L. bishopi
   L. geometricus
   L. mactans
Laugier's
   hernia
   sign

Launois-Cleret syndrome
Laurence-Biedl syndrome
Laurence-Moon-Biedl syndrome
Lawrence-Seip syndrome
LBBB (left bundle branch block)
LBF (Lactobacillus bulgaricus factor)
LCL (lymphocytic leukemia; lymphocytic lymphosarcoma)
LCM (lymphatic choriomeningitis)
LCM virus
LD (legionnaires' disease)
LE (lupus erythematosus)
Leber's optic atrophy
lechopyra
LED (lupus erythematosus disseminatus)
Lederer's anemia
Leeuwenhoekia australiensis
Legal's disease
Legg's disease
Legg-Calve-Perthes disease
Legionella
   L. bozemanii
   L. dumoffii
   L. feeleii
   L. gormanii
   L. jordanis
   L. longbeachae
   L. micdadei
   L. pittsburgensis
   L. pneumophila
   L. wadsworthii
legionella
legionellosis
legionnaires's disease
leiasthenia

Additional Entries

Leichtenstern's encephalitis
Leigh disease, syndrome
leiomyoblastoma
leiomyofibroma
leiomyoma
    bizarre l.
    l. cutis
    epithelioid l.
    l. uteri
    vascular l.
leiomyosarcoma
Leishmania
    L. aethiopica
    L. braziliensis
    L. caninum
    L. donovani
    L. farciminosa
    L. garnhami
    L. infantum
    L. major
    L. mexicana
    L. nilotica
    L. peruviana
    L. tropica
    L. tropica mexicana
leishmaniasis
    l. americana
    cutaneous l.
    diffuse cutaneous l.
    infantile l.
    lupoid l.
    mucocutaneous l.
    naso-oral l.
    nasopharyngeal l.
    post-kala-azar dermal l.
    l. recidivans l.
    l. tegmentaria diffusa
    visceral l.

lemoparalysis
lemostenosis
Lennert's lymphoma
Lennox syndrome
lentigo
    malignant l.
    nevoid l.
    senile l.
Lentivirinae
leontiasis
    l. ossea
Lepiota
    L. morgani
leprechaunism
leproma
leprosy
    l. bacillus
    borderline l.
    dimorphous l.
    intermediate l.
    lazarine l.
    lepromatous l.
    macular l.
    murine l.
    trophoneurotic l.
    tuberculoid l.
leptocytosis
leptodactyly
leptomeningioma
leptomeningitis
    l. interna
    sarcomatous l.
leptomeningopathy
Leptomitus
    L. epidermidis
    L. urophilus
    L. vaginae
Leptomonas

Additional Entries

leptonema
Leptopsylla
   L. segnis
Leptosphaeria
   L. senegalensis
Leptospira
   L. australis
   L. autumnalis
   L. biflexa
   L. canicola
   L. grippotyphosa
   L. hebdomidis
   L. hyos
   L. icterohaemorrhagiae
   L. interrogans
   L. pomona
leptospirosis
   anicteric l.
   benign l.
   l. icterohemorrhagica
leptospiruria
Leptothrix
Leptotrichia
   L. buccalis
   L. placoides
leptotrichosis
   l. conjunctivae
Leptrotrombidium
   L. akamushi
   L. deliense
Leptus
Leri's sign
Leriche's syndrome
Lermoyez's syndrome
Lesch-Nyhan syndrome
Leser-Trelat sign
lesion
   Armanni-Ebstein l.

lesion *(continued)*
   bird's nest l.
   Blumenthal l.
   Bracht-Wachter l.
   central l.
   coin l.
   Duret's l.
   Ebstein's l.
   Ghon's primary l.
   gross l.
   histologic l.
   impaction l.
   indiscriminate l.
   initial syphilitic l.
   irritative l.
   Janeway's l.
   jet l.
   Kimmelstiel-Wilson l.
   Lohlein-Baehr l.
   molecular l.
   onion scale l.
   organic l.
   peripheral l.
   precancerous l.
   primary l.
   ring-wall l.
   structural l.
   systemic l.
   total l.
   trophic l.
   wire-loop l.
Letterer-Siwe disease
Leudet's tinnitus
leukemia
   acute granulocytic l.
   acute lymphocytic l.
   acute megakaryoblastic l.
   acute monocytic l.

Additional Entries

leukemia *(continued)*
    acute myelogenous l.
    adult T-cell l.
    aleukemic granulocytic l.
    aleukemic lymphocytic l.
    aleukemic monocytic l.
    basophilic l.
    blast cell l.
    chronic granulocytic l.
    chronic lymphocytic l.
    chronic monocytic l.
    chronic myelocytic l.
    compound l.
    embryonal l.
    eosinophilic l.
    granulocytic l.
    Gross' l.
    hairy-cell l.
    hemoblastic l.,
        hemocytoblastic l.
    histiocytic l.
    lymphoblastic l.
    lymphocytic l.
    lymphosarcoma cell l.
    mast cell l.
    megakaryocytic l.
    micromyeloblastic l.
    monoblastic l.
    monocytic l.
    monomyelocytic l.
    myeloblastic l.
    myelocytic l.
    myelogenous l.
    myelomonocytic l.
    Naegeli type of monocytic l.
    plasmacytic l.
    promyelocytic l.

leukemia *(continued)*
    Rieder cell l.
    Schilling-type monocytic l.
    stem cell l.
    subleukemic granulocytic l.
    subleukemic lymphocytic l.
    subleukemic monocytic l.
    thrombocytic l.
    undifferentiated cell l.
leukemic
    l. reticuloendotheliosis
leukencephalitis
leukexosis
leukoblastosis
leukocythemia
leukocytoma
leukocytopenia
leukocytosis
    absolute l.
    agonal l.
    basophilic l.
    eosinophilic l.
    mononuclear l.
    neutrophilic l.
    pathologic l.
    physiologic l.
    pure l.
    relative l.
    terminal l.
    toxic l.
leukoderma
    l. acquisitum centrifugum
    l. colli
    occupational l.
    postinflammatory l.

Additional Entries

leukoderma *(continued)*
    syphilitic l.
leukodystrophy
    globoid l.
    hereditary cerebral l.
    Krabbe's l.
    metachromatic-type l.
    spongy degenerative-type l.
    sudanophilic l.
leukoedema
leukoencephalitis
    acute hemorrhagic l.
    l. periaxialis concentrica
    van Bogaert's sclerosing l.
leukoencephalopathy
    metachromatic l.
    progressive multifocal l.
    subacute sclerosing l.
leukoerythroblastic
    l. anemia
leukoerythroblastosis
leukokeratosis
leukolymphosarcoma
leukoma
    adherent l.
leukomyelitis
leukomyelopathy
leukomyoma
leukonecrosis
leukonychia
leukoparakeratosis
leukopathia
    l. punctata reticularis symmetrica
    l. unguium
leukopathy
leukopenia

leukopenia *(continued)*
    autoimmune l.
    basophilic l.
    congenital l.
    malignant l.
leukoplakia
    l. buccalis
    l. lingualis
    oral l.
    speckled l.
    l. vulvae
leukorrhagia
leukorrhea
leukosarcoma
leukosarcomatosis
leukosis
    acute l.
    lymphoid l.
    myeloblastic l.
    myelocytic l.
    skin l.
leukotaxis
leukovirus
Leyden's
    ataxia
    disease
Leyden-Mobius dystrophy
Leydig cell hyperplasia
Leydig-Sertoli cell tumor
LGB (Landry-Guillain-Barre syndrome)
LGV (lymphogranuloma venereum)
LIAFI (late infantile amaurotic familial idiocy)
Libman-Sacks endocarditis
lichen
    l. amyloidosus

Additional Entries

lichen *(continued)*
    l. corneus hypertrophicus
    l. myxedematosus
    l. nitidus
    l. obtusus corneus
    l. planus
    l. planus atrophicus
    l. planus erythematosus
    l. planus follicularis
    l. planus vesiculobullous
    l. ruber moniliformis
    l. sclerosus
    l. scrofulosus
    l. simplex chronicus
    l. spinulosus
    l. striatus
    l. tropicus
    l. urticatus
lichenoid
    l. dermatitis
        pigmented purpuric l. dermatitis
Lichtheimia corymbifera
Lichtheim's aphasia
Liepmann's apraxia
Limnatis
    L. granulosa
    L. mysomelas
    L. nilotica
Limulus
    L. polyphemus
Lindau's disease
Lindau-von Hippel disease
Linguatula
    L. serrata
linguatuliasis
linitis
    l. plastica

liparocele
lipedema
lipemia
    alimentary l.
    l. retinalis
lipid
    l. degeneration
    l. depletion
    l. disorder
    l. histiocytosis
    l. nephrosis
    l. pneumonia
    l. storage disease
lipidemia
lipidosis
    cerebroside l.
lipiduria
lipoadenoma
lipoarthritis
lipoatrophy
lipoblastomatosis
lipochondrodystrophy
lipochondroma
lipodystrophia
    l. intestinalis
    l. progressiva
lipodystrophy
    congenital progressive l.
    generalized l.
    inferior l.
    insulin l.
    intestinal l.
    partial l.
    progressive l.
lipofibroma
lipofuscinosis
    neuronal ceroid l.
lipogranuloma

Additional Entries

lipogranulomatosis
    Farber's l.
lipoid
    l. degeneration
    l. dystrophy
    l. granuloma
    l. nephrosis
    l. pneumonia
    l. proteinosis
lipoidosis
    arterial l.
    cerebroside l.
    cholesterol l.
    l. cutis et mucosae
    renal l.
lipoidproteinosis
lipoma
    l. annulare colli
    l. arborescens
    l. capsulare
    l. cavernosum
    diffuse l.
    l. diffusum renis
    l. dolorosa
    fetal l.
    fetal fat cell l.
    l. fibrosum
    intradural l.
    l. myxomatodes
    l. ossificans
    l. sarcomatodes
    telangiectatic l.
lipomatosis
    l. atrophicans
    congenital l. of pancreas
    l. dolorosa
    l. gigantea
    nodular circumscribed l.

lipomatosis *(continued)*
    renal l.
    symmetrical l.
lipomelanotic
    reticuloendothelial cell
    hyperplasia
lipomeningocele
lipomeria
lipomucopolysaccharidosis
lipomyohemangioma
lipomyoma
lipomyxoma
liponephrosis
lipopathy
lipopenia
lipophagia
    l. granulomatosis
lipoproteinemia
liposarcoma
Lipschutz ulcer
liquefactive
    l. degeneration
    l. necrosis
Lissauer's paralysis
Listeria
    L. monocytogenes
listeriosis
lithangiuria
lithiasis
    appendicular l.
    l. conjunctivae
    pancreatic l.
lithonephritis
lithureteria
Litten's sign
Little's disease
Littre's hernia
littritis

Additional Entries

liver
    albuminoid l.
    biliary cirrhotic l.
    brimstone l.
    l. cell adenoma
    l. cell carcinoma
    cirrhotic l.
    l. fluke
    frosted l.
    hobnail l.
    icing l.
    infantile l.
    iron l.
    lardaceous l.
    pigmented l.
    polycystic l.
    sago l.
    stasis l.
    sugar-icing l.
    waxy l.
livor mortis
LN (lipoid nephrosis; lupus nephritis)
lobar
    l. cerebral atrophy
    l. pneumonia
    l. pulmonary atrophy
lobomycosis
Lobo's disease
Lobstein's disease
lobster claw deformity
lobular
    l. adenocarcinoma
    l. carcinoma
    l. carcinoma, infiltrating
    l. carcinoma in situ
    l. glomerulonephritis
    l. pneumonia

lochiometritis
lochiorrhea
lockjaw
locomotor
    l. ataxia
Loffler's endocarditis
Lombardi's sign
Lorain's disease
lordoscoliosis
lordosis
lordotic
louping ill
    l. i. virus
louse (lice)
    body l.
    l.-borne typhus
    head l.
    pubic l.
lower
    l. nephron nephrosis
Lowe's syndrome
Lown-Gangong-Levine syndrome
Louis-Bar syndrome
loxarthron
loxarthrosis
Loxosceles
    L. laeta
    L. reclusa
loxoscelism
    viscerocutaneous l.
LS (lymphosarcoma)
LSA/RCS (lymphosarcoma-reticulum cell sarcoma)
LSM (late systolic murmur)
LTB (laryngotracheobronchitis)
Lucas' sign
Lucio leprosy

Additional Entries

Ludloff's sign
Ludwig's angina
lumbricosis
Lumbricus
lungworm
Lunyo virus
lupoid hepatitis
lupus
    chilblain l.
    drug-induced l.
    l. hypertrophicus
    laryngeal l.
    l. milaris disseminatus
      faciei
    neonatal l.
    l. nephritis
    l. pernio
    l. profundus
    l. tumidus
    l. vulgaris
lupus erythematosus
    acute disseminated l. e.
    cell l. e.
    chronic discoid l. e.
    l. e. cutaneous
    disseminated l. e.
    hypertrophic l. e.
    l. e. profundus
    l. e. tumidus
    systemic l. e.
luteal cyst
Lutembacher's syndrome
luteoma
LV (leukemia virus)
LVE (left ventricular enlargement)
LVF (left ventricular failure)
LVH (left ventricular hypertrophy)
lycopenemia
lycoperdonosis
Lyell's disease
Lyme disease
lymphadenectasis
lymphadenhypertrophy
lymphadenia
    l. ossea
lymphadenitis
    caseous l.
    dermatopathic l.
    mesenteric l.
    nonbacterial regional l.
    paratuberculous l.
    tuberculoid l
    tuberculous l.
lymphadenocele
lymphadenocyst
lymphadenoma
lymphadenopathy
    angioimmunoblastic l.
      with dysproteinemia
      (AILD)
    dermatopathic l.
    immunoblastic l.
    tuberculous l.
lymphadenosis
    aleukemic l.
    l. benigna cutis
lymphangiectasis
    intestinal l.
lymphangiitis
lymphangioendothelial sarcoma
lymphangioendothelioma
lymphangiofibroma
lymphangioma

Additional Entries

lymphangioma *(continued)*
   capillary l.
   l. cavernosum
   l. circumscriptum
   cystic l.
   fissural l.
   simple l.
lymphangiomyomatosis
lymphangiophlebitis
lymphangiosarcoma
lymphangitis
   l. carcinomatosa
   l. epizootica
   gummatous l.
   ulcerative l.
   l. ulcerosa pseudofarcinosa
lymphatitis
lymphedema
   congenital l.
   l. praecox
   l. tarda
lymphenteritis
lymphepithelioma
lymphnoditis
lymphoblastic
   l. leukemia
   l. lymphosarcoma
lymphoblastoma
lymphoblastosis
lymphocytapheresis
lymphocytic
   l. choriomeningitis
   l. choriomeningitis virus
   l. inflammatory infiltrate
   l. leukemia
   l. lymphoma
   l. lymphosarcoma

lymphocytic *(continued)*
   l. thyroiditis
lymphocytoma
   l. cutis
lymphocytopenia
lymphocytorrhexis
lymphocytosis
   acute infectious l.
   neutrophilic l.
lymphoepithelioma
lymphogranuloma
   l. inguinale
   l. malignum
   l. venereum
   l. venereum virus
lymphogranulomatosis
   benign l.
   l. cutis
   l. inguinalis
   l. maligna
lymphoid
   l. hyperplasia
   l. hypoplasia
   l. polyp
lymphoma
   African l.
   benign l.
   Burkitt's l.
   l. cutis
   diffuse l.
   follicular l.
   giant follicle l.
   granulomatous l.
   histiocytic l.
   Hodgkin's l.
   Lennert's l.
   lymphoblastic l.
   lymphocytic l.

Additional Entries

lymphoma *(continued)*
    lymphocytic l., poorly
        differentiated
    lymphocytic l., well-
        differentiated
    macrofollicular l.
    malignant l.,
        lymphosarcoma type
    Mediterranean l.
    mixed lymphocytic-
        histiocytic l.
    nodular l.
    non-Hodgkin's l.
    pleomorphic l.
    small B-cell l.
    stem cell l.
    T-cell l.'s
    T-cell l., convoluted
    T-cell l., cutaneous
    T-cell l., small
        lymphocytic
    U-cell l.
    undifferentiated l.
lymphomatoid
    l. granulomatosis
    l. papulosis
lymphomatosis
    neural l.
    occular l.
lymphomatous
lymphomyxoma
lymphopathia venereum
lymphopathy
    ataxic l.
lymphopenia
lymphoplasia
    cutaneous l.
lymphoproliferative syndrome
lymphoreticulosis
    benign l.
lymphorrhea
lymphorrhoid
lymphosarcoma
    cell leukemia l.
    fascicular l.
    lymphoblastic l.
    lymphocytic l.
    reticulum cell l.
    sclerosing l.
lymphosarcomatosis
lymphosporidiosis
lysosomal storage disease

Additional Entries

M

M (myopia)
M. (Micrococcus;
  Mycobacterium;
  Mycoplasma)
Mackenzie's disease
MacLean-Maxwell disease
MacLeod's syndrome
Macracanthorhynchus
  M. hirudinaceus
macroamylasemia
Macrobdella
macroblepharia
macrobrachia
macrocephaly
macrocheilia
macrocheiria
macrocnemia
macrocolon
macrocornea
macrocrania
macrocyst
macrocythemia
  hyperchromatic m.
macrocytic
  m. anemia
macrocytosis
macrodontia
macrodystrophia
  m. lipomatosa progressiva
macroesthesia
macrofollicular
  m. adenoma
  m. lymphoma
macrogenitosomia
macroglobulinemia

macroglobulinem *(continued)*
  Waldenstrom's m.
macroglossia
macrognathia
macrolymphocytosis
macromastia
macromelia
Macromonas
  M. bipunctata
  M. mobilis
Macrophoma
macrophthalmia
macrophthalmous
macroprolactinoma
macroprosopia
macrorhina
macroscelia
macrosigmoid
macrosomatia
  m. adiposa congenita
macrosomia
macrostomia
macular
  m. atrophy
  m. corneal dystrophy
  m. degeneration
  m. dysplasia
Madelung's deformity
Madurella
  M. grisea
  M. mycetomi
maduromycetoma
maduromycosis
maduromycotic mycetoma
maedivirus

Additional Entries

Maffucci's syndrome
Magendie-Hertwig sign
Magnan's sign
magnesemia
Maher's disease
Mahler's sign
Majocchi's
    disease
    granuloma
malabsorption syndrome
malacia
    metaplastic m.
    myeloplastic m.
    porotic m.
    m. traumatica
malacoplakia
    m. vesicae
malacosarcosis
maladie
    m. des jambes
    m. de plongeurs
    m. de Roger
    m. du sommeil
    m. des tics
malady
malaise
malakoplakia
malaria
    algid m.
    benign tertian m.
    bilious remittent m.
    bovine m.
    cerebral m.
    falciparum m.
    gastric m.
    hemolytic m.
    hemorrhagic m.
    induced m.

malaria *(continued)*
    malignant tertian m.
    ovale m.
    pernicious m.
    quartan m.
    quotidian m.
    subtertian m.
    tertian m.
    transfusion m.
    vivax m.
malarial
    m. nephropathy
    m. pigment deposition
Malassez's disease
Malassezia
    M. furfur
    M. macfadyani
    M. tropica
Malayan filariasis
male pseudohermaphroditism
male Turner's syndrome
    (Ullrich-Turner syndrome)
malformation
    Arnold-Chiari m.
    congenital m.
    Ebstein's m.
Malherbe's calcifying
    epithelioma
malignancy
malignant
    m. acanthosis nigricans
    m. adenoma
    m. disease
    m. edema
    m. exophthalmos
    m. freckle
    m. giant cell tumor of bone
    m. glaucoma

Additional Entries

malignant *(continued)*
   m. hypertension
   m. lymphocytoma
   m. lymphoma
   m. lymphoma,
      lymphosarcoma type
   m. melanoma
   m. meningioma
   m. mixed mesodermal
      tumor
   m. neoplasm
   m. pustule
   m. tumor
Malleomyces
   M. mallei
   M. pseudomallei
   M. whitmori
malleomycosis
Mallophaga
Mallory bodies
Mallory-Weiss syndrome
malnutrition
   malignant m.
   protein m.
malocclusion
     closed-bite m.
     open-bite m.
Malta fever (Brucellosis)
malum
   m. coxae
   m. coxae senilis
mamillitis
mammalgia
mammary
   m. duct ectasia
   m. dysplasia
   m. Paget's disease
mandibulofacial dysostosis

mange
Mann's sign
Mann-Williamson ulcer
Mannkopf's sign
mannosidosis
Manson's hemoptysis
Mansonella ozzardi
mansonelliasis
Mansonia
Mansonioides
manus
   m. cava
   m. curta
   m. extensa
   m. flexa
   m. valga
   m. vara
MAP (megaloblastic anemia of
   pregnancy)
maple syrup urine disease
marantic
   m. atrophy
   m. endocarditis
   m. thrombosis
   m. thrombus
marasmic kwashiokor
marasmus
marble bone disease
Marburg virus disease
marche a petits pas
Marchiafava-Bignami disease
Marchiafava-Micheli syndrome
Marfan's syndrome
margaritoma
marginal keratitis
Marie's disease
Marie-Bamberger disease
Marie-Strumpell disease

Additional Entries

Marie-Tooth disease
Marinesco's sign
Marituba virus
Marjolin's ulcer
Marochetti's blisters
Maroteaux-Lamy syndrome
Marsh's disease
maschaladenitis
masculinovoblastoma
Masson body
mastadenitis
mastadenoma
mastadenovirus
mastalgia
mastatrophy
mast cell
    m. c. hyperplasia
    m. c. leukemia
    m. c. sarcoma
    m. c. tumor
masthelcosis
mastitis
    chronic cystic m.
    fibrocystic m.
    gargantuan m.
    glandular m.
    interstitial m.
    m. neonatorum
    parenchymatous m.
    periductal m.
    phlegmonous m.
    plasma cell m.
    puerperal m.
    retromammary m.
    stagnation m.
    suppurative m.
mastocytoma
mastocytosis

mastodynia
mastoidalgia
mastoiditis
mastopathy
    fibrocystic m.
mastoplasia
Masugi-type nephrotoxic serum nephritis
mature
    m. abnormal chorion
    m. abnormal chorionic villi
    m. abnormal placenta
    m. cataract
maturity-onset diabetes
Mayaro virus
May-Hegglin anomaly
mazoplasia
MBD (Morquio-Brailsford disease)
MC (myocarditis)
McArdle-Schmid-Pearson disease
McArdle's syndrome
McCallum's plaque
M-component hypergammaglobulinemia
MCD (medullary cystic disease)
MCTD (mixed connective tissue disease)
MD (Marek's disease; muscular dystrophy; myocardial disease)
MDHV (Marek's herpesvirus disease)
MDUO (myocardial disease of unknown origin)

Additional Entries

MEA (multiple endocrine
  adenomatosis)
measles
    m. encephalitis
    German m. virus
    virus m.
mechanical ileus
Mecistocirrhus
Meckel's diverticulum
meconium
    m. extravasation
    m. peritonitis
    m. retention
medial
    m. arteriosclerosis
    m. cystic necrosis
    m. degeneration
    Monckeberg's m.
      calcification
    m. necrosis of aorta
median
    m. bar
    m. rhomboidal glossitis
mediastinal emphysema
mediastinitis
mediastinopericarditis
medina infection
medionecrosis
    m. aortae ediopathica
      cystica
    cystic m.
Mediterranean
    M. anemia
    M. fever
medullary
    m. adenocarcinoma
    m. carcinoma
    m. cystic disease of kidney

medullary *(continued)*
    m. fibrosarcoma
    m. histiocytic reticulosis
    m. necrosis
    m. reticulosis
    m. sponge kidney
    m. syndrome
medulloblastoma
medulloepithelioma
megacecum
megacolon
    aganglionic m.
    chronic idiopathic m.
    toxic m.
megacystis syndrome
megaduodenum
megaesophagus
megagnathus
megakaryocytic
    m. aplasia
    m. hyperplasia
    m. hypoplasia
    m. leukemia
    m. myelosis
megakaryocytosis
megakaryophthisis
megalencephaly
megaloblastic
    m. anemia
megaloblastosis
megalocardia
megalocephaly
megalocornea
megalocystis
megalogastria
megalomelia
megalonychosis
megalophthalmos

Additional Entries

megalosplanchnic
megaloureter
megaprosopous
Megaselia
Megasphaera
meibomianitis
meibomian
    m. cyst
Meig's syndrome
melalgia
melanoblastoma
melanocarcinoma
melanocytic
    m. nevus
melanocytoma
melanoderma
melanodermatitis
melanoepithelioma
melanoglossia
Melanoides
Melanolestes
    M. picipes
melanoma
    acral lentiginous m.
    amelanotic m.
    desmoplastic m.
    epithelioid cell m.
    juvenile m.
    lentigo maligna m.
    malignant m.
    nodular m.
    spindle cell m.
melanomatosis
melanonychia
melanoplakia
melanosarcoma
melanosis
    m. coli

melanosis *(continued)*
    Riehl's m.
    vagabond's m.
melanotic
    m. freckle of Hutchinson
    m. progonoma
    m. sarcoma
    m. whitlow
melanuria
melena
melioidosis
melitis
melituria
    glycosuric m.
    m. inosita
    nondiabetic glycosuric m.
Melkersson's syndrome
Melkersson-Rosenthal
    syndrome
Meloidogyne
    M. javanica
melomelus
melorheostosis
melotus
membrane
    acute inflammatory m.
    acute pyogenic m.
    diphtheritic m.
    inflammatory m.
membranoproliferative
    glomerulonephritis
membranous
    m. acute inflammation
    m. cataract
    m. glomerulonephritis
    m. nephropathy
MEN (multiple endocrine
    neoplasia)

Additional Entries

Mendelson's syndrome
Menetrier's disease
Mengo virus
Meniere's disease
meningeal
    m. sarcoma
    m. sarcomatosis
meningioma
    angiomatous m.
    fibroblastic m.
    malignant m.
    meningothelial m.
    psammomatous m.
meningiomatosis
    diffuse m.
meningitis
    amebic m.
    aseptic m.
    bacterial m.
    cryptococcal m.
    meningococcal m.
    mycotic m.
    pyogenic m.
    syphilitic m.
    torular m.
    tuberculous m.
    viral m.
meningoarteritis
meningocele
meningocerebritis
meningococcemia
meningococcin
meningococcus
meningoencephalitis
meningoencephalocele
meningoencephalomyelitis
meningoencephalopathy
    carcinomatous m.

meningomyelitis
meningomyelocele
meningomyeloradiculitis
meningopneumonitis
meningothelial meningioma
Menkes' syndrome
menometrorrhagia
menoplania
menorrhagia
menostaxis
meralgia
    m. paresthetica
meromelia
Merzbacher-Pelizaeus disease
mesangial
    m. proliferative
        glomerulopathy
mesencephalitis
mesenchymal tumor
mesenchymoma
mesenteric
    m. cyst
    m. hyperplasia
    m. lymphadenitis
    m. thrombosis
mesenteritis
mesoappendicitis
mesobacterium
mesoblastic nephroma
Mesocestoides
    M. variabilis
mesonephric
    m. adenocarcinoma
    m. cyst
mesonephroma
    m. ovarii
mesothelial
    m. cyst

Additional Entries

mesothelial *(continued)*
    m. sarcoma
mesothelioma
    fibrous m.
metabolic
    m. acidosis
    m. alkalosis
    m. craniopathy
    m. ileus
    m. insufficiency
metachromasia
metachromatic leukodystrophy
metagonimiasis
Metagonimus
    M. ovatus
    M. yokogawai
metaphyseal
    m. chondrodysplasia
    m. dysostosis
    m. dysplasia
metaphysitis
metaplasia
    agnogenic myeloid m.
    apocrine m.
    cartilaginous m.
    chondroid m.
    decidual m.
    endothelial m.
    epidermoid m.
    glandular m.
    Hurthle cell m.
    intestinal m.
    myeloid m.
    osseous m.
    squamous m.
metaplastic keratinization
metastasizing struma
metastatic

metastatic *(continued)*
    m. abscess
    m. calcification
    m. carcinoma
    m. neoplasm
    m. ophthalmia
    m. parotitis
    m. tumor
Metastrongylus
    M. elongatus
metatarsalgia
metatarsus
    m. abductus
    m. adductus
meteorism
Methanobacterium
Methanococcus
methemoglobinemia
    hereditary enzymatic-type m.
methionine malabsorption syndrome
metritis
metrocele
metrocolpocele
metrocystosis
metromalacia
metropathy
metrophlebitis
metroptosis
metrorrhagia
metrorrhexis
metrosalpingitis
metrostaxis
metrostenosis
MF (mycosis fungoides)
MG (myasthenia gravis)

Additional Entries

MGN (membranous
　　glomerulonephritis)
mgtis (meningitis)
MHA (microangiopathic
　　hemolytic anemia)
Michaelis-Gutmann bodies
Mibelli's porokeratosis
microabscess
　　Munro m.
　　Pautrier m.
microaerophilic
　　m. streptococcus
microaneurysm
microangiopathic
　　m. hemolytic anemia
microangiopathy
　　diabetic m.
　　thrombotic m.
Microbacterium
Micrococcus
　　M. flavus
　　M. intracellularis
　　M. pyogenes var. aureus
　　M. tetragenus
microcythemia
microcytic
　　m. anemia
　　m. hypochromic anemia
microcytosis
microdrepanocytic disease
Microfilaria
　　M. bancrofti
　　M. streptocerca
microfilariasis
microfollicular adenoma
microglioma
microgliomatosis
microglossia

micrognathia
microinvasive carcinoma
microlithiasis
micromelia
Micromonospora
　　M. faeni
microscopic infarct
microspherocytosis
Microsporon
microsporosis
Microsporum
　　M. audouini
　　M. canis
　　M. felineum
　　M. ferrugineum
　　M. fulvum
　　M. furfur
　　M. gypseum
　　M. lanosum
　　M. nanum
microstomia
middle lobe syndrome
midline
　　m. lethal granuloma
midzonal necrosis
Miescheria
migraine
migrating thrombophlebitis
Mikulicz's disease
miliaria
　　m. profunda
　　m. pustulosa
　　m. rubra
miliary
　　m. abscess
　　m. aneurysm
　　m. granulomatous
　　　　inflammation

Additional Entries

miliary *(continued)*
    m. tuberculosis
milium cyst
milk
    m. alkali syndrome
    biundulant m. fever
Milkman's syndrome
Milroy's disease
Mima
    M. polymorpha
Minimata disease
minuthesis
miosis
mite
    parasitoid m.
    red m.
    trombiculid m.
mitochondrial myopathy
mitral
    m. regurgitation
    m. stenosis
    m. valve calcification
    m. valve prolapse
mixed
    m. connective tissue disease
    m. tumor
Miyagawanella
    M. illinii
    M. louisianae
    M. lymphogranulomatosis
    M. ornithosis
    M. pneumoniae
    M. psittaci
MLA (monocytic leukemia, acute)
MLC (myelomonocytic leukemia, chronic)
MLS (myelomonocytic leukemia, subacute)
MLV (Moloney's leukemogenic virus)
MM (malignant melanoma; mutliple myeloma; myeloid metaplasia)
MMM (myeloid metaplasia with myelofibrosis; myelosclerosis with myeloid metaplasia)
MMTV (mouse mammary tumor virus)
Moberg's arthrodesis
Mobius' disease
mole
    Breus m.
    hydatid m.
    hydatidiform m.
    invasive m.
Moloney's
    leukemogenic virus
    sarcoma virus
monarthritis
Monckeberg's
    arteriosclerosis
    medial calcification
Mondor's disease
Monge's disease
mongolian idiot
mongolism
mongoloid
Monilia
    M. sitophila
moniliasis
Moniliformia
    M. moniliformis
monoblastic leukemia

Additional Entries

monocytic
    m. inflammatory infiltrate
    m. leukemia
monocytopenia
monocytosis
monomyelocytic leukemia
monomyositis
Mononchus
mononeuritis
    m. multiplex
mononeuropathy
mononucleosis
    infectious m.
monoplegia
Monosporium
    M. apiospermum
monostotic fibrous dysplasia
Monotrichia
Monro's abscesses
Morax-Axenfeld
    bacillus
    diplococcus
    hemophilus
Moraxella
    M. kingae
    M. lacunata
    M. liquefaciens
    M. lwoffi
    M. nonliquefaciens
    M. osloensis
    M. phenylpyruvica
    M. urethralis
morbillivirus
Morgagni's
    cyst
    hernia
    syndrome
Morganella

Morganella *(continued)*
    M. morganii
Morgan's bacillus
Morquio-Brailsford disease
Morquio's disease
Morton's
    disease
    neuralgia
motor aphasia
MPGN (membranoproliferative glomerulonephritis)
MR (mitral regurgitation)
MS (multiple sclerosis)
MSUD (maple syrup urine disease)
MSV (Moloney's sarcoma virus)
MT (malignant teratoma)
MTI (malignant teratoma intermediate)
MTT (malignant trophoblastic teratoma)
mucinosis
mucinous
    m. adenocarcinoma
    m. atrophy
    m. carcinoma
    m. cyst
    m. cystadenocarcinoma
    m. cystadenoma
    m. degeneration
mucocele
mucoenteritis
mucoepidermoid
    m. carcinoma
    m. tumor
mucolipidosis
mucopolysaccharidosis
mucopurulent exudate

Additional Entries

Mucor
- M. corymbifer
- M. mucedo
- M. pusillus
- M. racemosus
- M. ramosus
- M. rhizopodiformis

Mucoraceae
mucormycosis
mucosal neuroma syndrome
mucous
- m. colitis
- m. cyst
- m. plug

mucoviscidosis
mullerian tumor
Multiceps
- M. glomeratus
- M. multiceps
- M. serialis

multifocal
- m. fibrosis
- m. inflammation
- m. progressive leukoencephalopathy

multilocular cyst
multiple
- m. adenomatous polyps
- m. endocrine neoplasia
- m. hemorrhagic sarcoma
- m. meningiomas
- m. myeloma
- m. neurofibromatosis
- m. sclerosis

Munchausen's syndrome
Munro microabscess
mural thrombosis
murine typhus

murmur
- aortic m.
- apical m.
- Austin Flint m.
- basal m.
- cardiac m.
- cardiovascular m.
- continuous m.
- diastolic m.
- ejection m.
- holosystolic m.
- regurgitant m.
- systolic m.
- venous m.
- ventricular filling m.
- vescicular m.

Murray Valley encephalitis virus
Musca
- M. domestica
- M. volitans

muscular atrophy
- Charcot-Marie-Tooth m. a.
- hypertrophic polyneuritic-type m. a.
- infantile m.a.
- peroneal m. a.
- progressive m. a.

muscular dystrophy
- distal-type m. d.
- Duchenne-type m. d.
- facioscapulohumeral-type m.d.
- Landouzy-Dejerine progressive m. d.
- limb girdle-type m. d.
- ophthalmoplegic-type m. d.

Additional Entries

musculoaponeurotic
   fibromatosis
My (myopia)
myalgia
myasthenia gravis
myatrophy
Mycelia
   M. sterilia
mycetoma
mycetosis
mycobacteria
   anonymous m.
   atypical m.
   Group I-IV m.
   nonphotochromogenic m.
   photochromogenic m.
   scotochromogenic m.
mycobacteriosus
Mycobacterium
   M. abscessus
   M. aquae
   M. balnei
   M. berolinenis
   M. borstelense
   M. bovis
   M. butyricum
   M. chelonei
   M. flavescens
   M. fortuitum
   M. gastri
   M. gordonae
   M. habana
   M. haemophilum
   M. intracellularis
   M. johnei
   M. kansasii
   M. leprae
   M. leprae murium

Mycobacterium *(continued)*
   M. luciflavum
   M. malmoense
   M. marinum
   M. microti
   M. nonchromogenicum
   M. paratuberculosis
   M. peregrinum
   M. phlei
   M. scrofulaceum
   M. simiae
   M. smegmatis
   M. szulgai
   M. terrea-nonchromogenicum-triviale
   M. triviale
   M. tuberculosis
   M. tuberculosis var. avium
   M. tuberculosis var. hominis
   M. tuberculosis var. muris
   M. ulcerans
   M. xenopi
mycobacterium
Mycocandida
Mycococcus
Mycoderma
   M. aceti
   M. dermatitidis
   M. immite
mycomyringitis
Mycoplana
   M. bullata
   M. dimorpha
Mycoplasma
   M. buccale

Additional Entries

Mycoplasma *(continued)*
    M. faucium
    M. fermentans
    M. hominis
    M. orale
    M. pharyngis
    M. pneumoniae
    M. salivarium
mycosis fungoides
mycotic
    m. aneurysm
    m. keratitis
mycotoxicosis
mydriasis
myelin degeneration
myelitis
    transverse m.
myeloblastic leukemia
myelocele
myelocystocele
myelocystomeningocele
myelocytic leukemia
myeloencephalitis
myelofibrosis
myelogenous leukemia
myeloid
    m. hyperplasia
    m. metaplasia
    m. metaplasia, agnogenic
myelolipoma
myeloma
    plasma cell m.
    plasmacytic m.
myelomalacia
myelomatosis
myelomeningitis
myelomeningocele
myelomonocytic leukemia

myelopathy
    transverse m.
myelophthisis
myeloradiculitis
myelorrhagia
myelosarcoma
myeloschisis
myelosclerosis
myelosis
    aleukemic m.
    erythremic m.
    megakaryocytic m.
    nonleukemic m.
myelosyringosis
myiasis
myoblastoma
    granular cell m.
myocardial
    m. infarct
    m. infarction
    m. ischemia
myocarditis
    Fiedler's m.
    Loffler's m.
    rheumatic m.
myoclonic epilepsy
myoepithelioma
myofibroma
myofibrosis
myofibrositis
myoglobinemia
myoglobinuria
    acute paroxysmal m.
myoglobinuric nephrosis
myolipoma
myoma
myomalacia
myometritis

Additional Entries

myonecrosis
myopathy
    alcoholic m.
    congenital m.
    corticosteroid m.
    endocrine m.
    nemaline m.
myopericarditis
myopia
myorrhexis
myosarcoma
myosis
    endolymphatic stromal m.
myositis
    clostridial m.
    m. ossificans
    m. ossificans progressiva
    ossifying interstitial m.
myotonia
    m. acquisita
    m. atrophica
    m. congenita
    m. dystrophica
    m. neonatorum
myotonic dystophy
myringitis
    bullous m.
myringomycosis
Myrotophyllum
    M. hepatis
myxadenitis

myxedema
    m. coma
    pituitary m.
    pretibial m.
myxochondroma
myxofibroma
myxofibrosarcoma
myxoid
    m. cyst
    m. degeneration
    m. fibroma
myxolipoma
myxoliposarcoma
myxoma
    atrial m.
    cardiac m.
    cystic m.
    endochondromatous m.
    erectile m.
    infectious m.
    lipomatous m.
    odontogenic m.
    vascular m.
myxomatosis
    cardiac valve m.
myxomatous degeneration
myxopapillary ependymoma
myxosarcoma
myxovirus
Myzomyia
Myzorhynchus

Additional Entries

Additional Entries

N

N. (Neisseria; Nocardia)
nabothian cyst
Naegeli type of monocytic
    leukemia
Naegeli's
    leukemia
    syndrome
Naegleria
naegleriasis
Naffziger's syndrome
nail-patella syndrome
nanism
    mulibrey n.
    pituitary n.
    renal n.
    senile n.
    symptomatic n.
nanophthalmos
Nannizzia
    N. cajetani
    N. grubia
    N. gypsea
    N. incurvata
    N. obtusa
narcolepsy
narcosis
    basal n.
    carbon dioxide n.
    insufflation n.
    intravenous n.
    medullary n.
    nitrogen n.
    Nussbaum's n.
nasal
    n. glioma

nasal *(continued)*
    n. lymphoepithelioma
    n. plasmacytoma
    n. polyp
nasopharyngitis
nasoseptitis
nasosinusitis
natriuresis
nausea
    n. epidemica
    n. gravidarum
NBTE (nonbacterial thrombotic
    endocarditis)
NCA (neurocirculatory asthenia)
ND (neonatal death; Newcastle
    disease)
NDI (nephrogenic diabetes
    insipidus)
NDV (Newcastle disease virus)
nearsightedness
Necator
    N. americanus
necatoriasis
Necrobacterium necrophorum
necrobiosis
    n. lipoidica diabeticorum
necrophagocytosis
necrosis
    acute inflammatory n.
    aseptic n.
    avascular n.
    caseous n.
    central n.
    centrilobular n.
    cerebrocortical n.

Additional Entries

necrosis *(continued)*
    cheesy n.
    coagulative n.
    cortical n.
    cystic medial n.
    cytodegenerative n.
    cytotoxic n.
    diffuse n
    epiphyseal ischemic n.
    Erheim's cystic medial n.
    exanthematous n.
    fat n.
    fibrinoid n.
    focal n.
    gangrenous n.
    hyaline n.
    inflammatory n.
    ischemic n.
    lamellar n.
    liquefactive n.
    massive hepatic n.
    medial n.
    medullary n.
    midzonal n.
    Paget's quiet n.
    papillary n.
    peripheral n.
    periportal n.
    postpartum pituitary n.
    radiation n.
    radium n.
    renal medullary n.
    renal papillary n.
    sclerosing n.
    septic n.
    tumor n.
    Zenker's n.
    zonal n.

necrotic
necrotizing
    n. angiitis
    n. arteriolitis
    n. bronchopneumonia
    n. glomerulonephritis
    n. inflammation
    n. lobar pneumonia
    n. pancreatitis
    n. papillitis
    n. vasculitis
NED (no evidence of disease)
Neisseria
    N. catarrhalis
    N. caviae
    N. flava
    N. flavescens
    N. gonorrhoeae
    N. intracellularis
    N. lactamicus
    N. meningitidis
    N. mucosa
    N. ovis
    N. perflava
    N. pharyngis
    N. sicca
    N. subflava
Neisser
    diplococcus of N.
Nelson's syndrome
Nemathelminthes
nematosis
neoplasia
    multiple endocrine n.
neoplasm
    adrenal n.
    benign n.
    epithelial n.

Additional Entries

neoplasm *(continued)*
    malignant n.
    metastatic n.
neoplastic
nephritis
    acute n.
    arteriosclerotic n.
    azotemic n.
    bacterial n.
    Balkan n.
    capsular n.
    caseous n.
    chronic n.
    congenital n.
    degenerative n.
    n. dolorosa
    exudative n.
    fibrolipomatous n.
    fibrous n.
    glomerular n.
    glomerulocapsular n.
    n. gravidarum
    hemorrhagic n.
    indurative n.
    interstitial n.
    intestinal n.
    Lancereaux's n.
    lipomatous n.
    lupus n.
    Masugi-type nephrotoxic
        serum n.
    parenchymatous n.
    pneumococcus n.
    potassium-losing n.
    n. of pregnancy
    productive n.
    n. repens
    salt-losing n.

nephritis *(continued)*
    scarletinal n.
    suppurative n.
    syphilitic n.
    tartrate n.
    transfusion n.
    tubular n.
    tuberculous n.
    vascular n.
nephroangiosclerosis
nephroblastoma
nephrocalcinosis
nephrocele
nephrocoloptosis
nephrocystitis
nephrocystosis
nephrohemia
nephrohypertrophy
nephrolithiasis
nephroma
    embryonal n.
    mesoblastic n.
nephromalacia
nephronophthisis
    familial juvenile n.
nephropathy
    acute uric acid n.
    analgesic n.
    Balkan n.
    diabetic n.
    gouty n.
    hemoglobinuric n.
    IgA n.
    membranous n.
    myoglobinuric n.
    reflux n.
    sickle cell n.
    tubulointerstitial n.

Additional Entries

nephroptosis
nephropyelitis
nephropyosis
nephrorrhagia
nephrosclerosis
   arteriolar n.
   benign n.
   hyaline n.
   hyperplastic n.
   intercapillary n.
   malignant n.
   senile n.
nephrosis
   acute n.
   amyloid n.
   bile n.
   cholemic n.
   chronic n.
   Epstein's n.
   hemoglobinuric n.
   hypokalemic n.
   lipid n.
   lipoid n.
   lower nephron n.
   myoglobinuric n.
   necrotizing n.
   osmotic n.
   toxic n.
   tubular n.
   vacuolar n.
nephrosonephritis
   hemorrhagic n.
nephrotic syndrome
nephrotoxic serum nephritis, Masugi type
nephrotoxin
nephrotuberculosis
neuralgia

neuralgia *(continued)*
   cardiac n.
   cervicobrachial n.
   cervico-occipital n.
   cranial n.
   geniculate n.
   glossopharyngeal n.
   idiopathic n.
   intercostal n.
   mammary n.
   mandibular joint n.
   migrainous n.
   Morton's n.
   nasociliary n.
   peripheral n.
   postherpetic n.
   sphenopalatine n.
   stump n.
   supraorbital n.
   trifacial n.
   trigeminal n.
   vidian n.
   visceral n.
neuralgic
   n. amyotrophy
neurapraxia
neurasthenia
neurilemmitis
neurilemoma
   ameloblastic n.
   malignant n.
neurilemosarcoma
neurinoma
neuritic atrophy
neuritis
neuroarthropathy
neuroastrocytoma
neuroblastoma

Additional Entries

neuroblastoma *(continued)*
    olfactory n.
neurochoroiditis
neurocirculatory asthenia
neurocytoma
neurodermatitis
neurocephalomyelopathy
neuroepithelioma
neurofibroma
    plexiform n.
neurofibromatosis
neurofibrosarcoma
neurogenic
    n. bladder
    n. sarcoma
neuroleptanalgesia
neuroleptanesthesia
neuroleptic
neuroma
    acoustic n.
    amputation n.
    mucosal n.
    plexiform n.
    traumatic n.
neuromalacia
neuromyelitis
    n. optica
neuromyositis
neuromyotonia
neuronevus
neuronophagia
neuroparalysis
neuropathology
neuropathy
    amblyopia n.
    amyloid n.
    diabetic n.
    entrapment n.

neuropathy *(continued)*
    hereditary sensory
        radicular n.
    hypertrophic interstitial n.
    peripheral n.
    retrobulbar n.
    vincristine n.
neuroretinitis
neuroretinopathy
neurosarcoma
neurosclerosis
neurosis
    anxiety n.
    compensation n.
    obsessive-compulsive n.
    phobic n.
Neurospora
    N. sitophilia
neurosyphilis
neutropenia
neutrophilic
    n. hyperplasia
    n. infiltrate
    n. leukemia
    n. leukocytosis
nevocarcinoma
nevoxanthoendothelioma
nevus
    araneus n.
    bathing trunk n.
    blue n.
    cellular blue n.
    compound n.
    dermal n.
    dermal-epidermal n.
    epithelioid n.
    n. flammeus
    giant blue n.

Additional Entries

nevus *(continued)*
    intradermal n.
    intraepidermal n.
    Jadassohn's n.
    junctional n.
    lymphatic n.
    melanocytic n.
    nevocytic n.
    pigmented n.
    sebaceous n.
    spider n.
    spindle cell n.
    Spitz n.
    spongy n.
    n. unius lateris
    vascular n.
newborn
    n. hemolytic disease
    n. hemorrhagic disease
    icterus gravis of n.
    n. respiratory syndrome
Newcastle disease
Newcastle disease virus
Newcastle-Manchester bacillus
New World hookworm
NGU (nongonococcal urethritis)
NHA (nonspecific hepatocellular abnormality)
Nicollella
NIDDM (noninsulin-dependent diabetes mellitus)
Niemann-Pick disease
Nikolsky's sign
Nitrobacter
Nitrocystis
NLA (neuroleptanalgesia)
NMA (neurogenic muscular atrophy)

Nocardia
    N. asteroides
    N. brasiliensis
    N. caviae
    N. madurae
    N. minutissima
    N. pelletieri
    N. tenuis
nocardiosis
Nocard's bacillus
nocturia
nocturnal
    n. dyspnea
    n. hemoglobinuria
nodular
    n. calcific aortic stenosis
    n. calcific stenosis
    n. colloid goiter
    n. fibrosis
    n. glomerulosclerosis
    n. goiter
    n. hidradenoma
    n. hyperplastic goiter
    n. lymphoma
    n. nonsuppurative panniculitis
    n. vasculitis
Noguchia
    N. granulosus
nonchromaffin paraganglioma
noncommunicating hydrocephalus
nongonococcal urethritis
noninsulin-dependent diabetes mellitus
Nonne's syndrome
Nonne-Milroy-Meige syndrome
Noonan's syndrome

Additional Entries

normoblastosis
normocalcemia
normocytosis
normoglycemia
normokalemia
normo-orthocytosis
Norrie's disease
North American blastomycosis
Norum's disease
Norwalk virus
nosomycosis
Nosopsyllus
    N. fasciatus
nosotoxicosis
notencephalocele
NPD (Niemann-Pick disease)
NS (nephrotic syndrome)
NSU (nonspecific urethritis)
Ntaya virus
nuchal
    n. hemangioma
    n. rigidity
NUG (necrotizing ulcerative gingivitis)
Nussbaum's narcosis
NVD (Newcastle virus disease)
nyctalopia
Nygmia
Nyssorhynchus
nystagmus
    amaurotic n.
    amblyopic n.
    ataxic n.
    aural n.
    caloric n.
    central n.
    Cheyne's n.

nystagmus *(continued)*
    congenital n.
    convergence n.
    disjunctive n.
    dissociated n.
    downbeat n.
    electrical n.
    end-position n.
    fixation n.
    gaze n.
    jerky n.
    labyrinthine n.
    latent n.
    lateral n.
    miner's n.
    ocular n.
    opticokinetic n.
    oscillating n.
    palatal n.
    paretic n.
    pendular n.
    periodic alternating n.
    positional n.
    resilient n.
    retraction n.
    rotary n.
    secondary n.
    see-saw n.
    spontanous n.
    undulatory n.
    unilateral n.
    vertical n.
    vestibular n.
    vibratory n.
    visual n.
    voluntary n.

Additional Entries

Additional Entries

O

OA (osteoarthritis)
OAD (obstructive airway disease)
OAP (osteoarthropathy)
oasthouse urine disease
oat cell
    o. c. carcinoma
OAV (oculoauriculovertebral dysplasia)
obesity
    adult-onset o.
    alimentary o.
    endogenous o.
    exogenous o.
    hyperinterrenal o.
    hyperplasmic o.
    hypertrophic o.
    life-long o.
    morbid o.
    simple o.
obliterative
    o. endocarditis
    o. inflammation
    o. pleuritis
OBS (organic brain syndrome)
obsessive-compulsive
    o.-c. neurosis
    o.-c. psychoneurosis
obstruction
    complete o.
    intestinal o.
    mesenteric vascular o.
    partial o.
    urinary o.
obstructive

obstructive *(continued)*
    o. cirrhosis
    o. diverticulitis
    o. emphysema
    o. hyperbilirubinuria
    o. jaundice
    o. pulmonitis
occupational lung disease
Ochromyia
    O. anthropophaga
ochronosis
    exogenous o.
    ocular o.
Octomitus
    O. hominis
oculomycosis
ODD (oculodentodigital dysplasia)
odontogenic
    o. cyst
    o. fibroma
    o. fibrosarcoma
    o. myxoma
    o. tumor
odontoma
    ameloblastic o.
    complex o.
    compound o.
    fibroameloblastic o.
odynophagia
Oehler's symptom
Oesophagostomum
    O. apiostomum
    O. bifurcum
    O. stephanostomum

Additional Entries

Oestrus
    O. hominis
    O. ovis
Oguchi's disease
oidiomycosis
OKN (optokinetic nystagmus)
Old World hookworm
olecranarthropathy
oligemia
oligocythemia
oligdactyly
oligodendroblastoma
oligodendroglia
oligodendroglioma
    Grade I
    Grades II-IV
oligohydramnios
oligomenorrhea
oligophrenia
    phenylpyruvic o.
oliguria
Oliver's sign
olivocerebellar atrophy
olivopontocerebellar atrophy
Ollier's disease
OM (otitis media)
OMD (ocular muscle dystrophy)
OMI (old myocardial infarction)
omphalelcosis
omphalitis
omphalocele
omphaloma
omphalophlebitis
omphalorrhagia
omphalorrhexis
Omsk hemorrhagic fever
Onchocerca
    O. caecutiens

Onchocerca *(continued)*
    O. cervicalis
    O. lienalis
    O. volvulus
onchocerciasis
onchocercoma
oncocytic adenoma
oncocytoma
oncoma
Oncomelania
oncornavirus
oncosis
oncothlipsis
onychatrophia
onychomalacia
onychomycosis
onychorrhexis
O'nyong-nyong fever
O'nyong-nyong fever virus
oophoritis
    o. parotidea
oophorocystosis
oophoroma
    o. folliculare
oophoropathy
oophorosalpingitis
oophorrhagia
Oospora
opalgia
open spina bifida
ophiasis
ophthalmagra
ophthalmalgia
ophthalmatrophia
ophthalmia
    catarrhal o.
    o. eczematosa
    Egyptian o.

Additional Entries

ophthalmia *(continued)*
    gonococcal o.
    gonorrheal o.
    granular o.
    hepatic o.
    metastatic o.
    migratory o.
    mucous o.
    o. neonatorum
    neuroparalytic o.
    o. nivialis
    o. nodosa
    periodic o.
    purulent o.
    scrofulous o.
    o. sympathetic
    transferred o.
    varicose o.
ophthalmitis
    sympathetic o.
ophthalmoblennorrhea
ophthalmocele
ophthalmodesmitis
ophthalodonesis
ophthalmolith
ophthalmomalacia
ophthalmomycosis
ophthalmomyiasis
ophthalmomyitis
ophthalmomyositis
ophthalmoneuritis
ophthalmoneuromyelitis
ophthalmopathy
    external o.
    infiltrative o.
    internal o.
ophthalmoplegia
    basal o.

ophthalmoplegia *(continued)*
    exophthalmic o.
    external o.
    fascicular o.
    internal o.
    internuclear o.
    nuclear o.
    orbital o.
    Parinaud's o.
    partial o.
    progressive external o.
ophthalmoplegic-type
    progressive muscular
    dystrophy
ophthalmorrhagia
ophthalmorrhea
ophthalmorrhexis
ophthalmosynchysis
opisthorchiasis
Opisthrochis
    O. felineus
    O. noverca
    O. viverrini
opisthorchosis
Opitz's disease
Oppenheim's disease
opportunistic infection
orbivirus
orchiditis
orchidoncus
orchidoptosis
orchiencephaloma
orchiepididymitis
orchiocele
orchiomyeloma
orchioncus
orchioneuralgia
orchiopathy

Additional Entries

orchioscheocele
orchioscirrhus
orchitis
    autoimmune o.
    granulomatous o.
    metastatic o.
    spermatogenic
        granulomatous o.
    traumatic o.
    o. variolosa
orf virus
organized
    o. hematoma
    o. pneumonia
    o. thrombus
Oriboca virus
oriental
    o. body fluke
    o. lung fluke
    o. sore
Ormond's disease
orofaciodigital syndrome
orogenital syndrome
Oropouche virus
Oroya fever
orthomyxovirus
orthopnea
orthopoxvirus
orthostatic
    o. albuminuria
    o. hypertension
    o. hypotension
Osgood-Schlatter disease
Osler's
    disease
    erythema
Osler-Vaquez disease
Osler-Weber-Rendu disease

osmotic nephrosis
osseous metaplasia
ossifying
    o. fibroma
    o. inflammation
    o. interstitial myositis
ostealgia
osteitis
    acute o.
    o. condensans
    o. deformans
    o. fibrosa cystica
    o. fibrosa disseminata
    necrotic o.
    parathyroid o.
    productive o.
    sarcomatous o.
    sclerosing o.
    secondary hyperplastic o.
    vascular o.
osteoarthritis
    o. deformans
    hyperplastic o.
    interphalangeal o.
osteoarthropathy
    familial o. of fingers
    hypertrophic o., idiopathic
    hypertrophic o., primary
    hypertrophic pneumic o.
    hypertrophic pulmonary o.
    pulmonary o.
    secondary hypertrophic o.
osteoarthrosis
osteoblastoma
osteocachexia
osteocampsia
osteocartilaginous exostosis
osteocele

Additional Entries

osteochondritis
    calcaneal o.
    o. deformans juvenilis
    o. dissecans
    o. ischiopubica
    o. necroticans
    o. ossis metacarpi et
        metatarsi
osteochondrodysplasia
osteochondrodystrophy
    familial o.
osteochondrofibroma
osteochondroma
    fibrosing o.
osteochondromatosis
    synovial o.
osteochondromyxoma
osteochondropathy
    polyglucose sulfate-
        induced o.
osteochondrosarcoma
osteochondrosis
    o. deformans biae
osteoclasia
osteoclastoma
osteocystoma
osteodynia
osteodysplasty
    o. of Melnick and Needles
osteodystrophy
    Albright's hereditary o.
    renal o.
osteoectasia
    familial o.
osteoenchondroma
osteofibrochondrosarcoma
osteofibroma
osteofibromatosis

osteofibromatos *(continued)*
    cystic o.
osteogenic sarcoma
osteohalisteresis
osteohemachromatosis
osteohydatidosis
osteolathyrism
osteolipochondroma
osteolipoma
osteoma
    compact o.
    o. cutis
    fibrous o.
    giant osteoid o.
    parosteal o.
    o. sarcomatosus
    o. spongiosum
osteomalacia
    hepatic o.
    infantile o.
    osteogenic o.
    puerperal o.
    renal tubular o.
    senile o.
osteomiosis
oeteomyelitis
    conchiolin o.
    Garre's sclerosing o.
    malignant o.
    pyogenic o.
    salmonella o.
    sclerosing nonsuppurative
        o.
    tuberculous o.
    typhoid o.
    o. variolosa
osteomyelodysplasia
osteomyelosclerosis

Additional Entries

osteomyxochondroma
osteonecrosis
osteoneuralgia
osteopathia
osteopathy
    alimentary o.
    disseminated condensing o.
    myelogenic o.
osteoperiostitis
osteopetrosis
osteophlebitis
osteophyma
osteopoikilosis
osteoporosis
    o. circumscripta
    o. of disuse
    postmenopausal o.
    post-traumatic o.
    senile o.
osteopsathyrosis
osteorrhagia
osteosarcoma
    parosteal o.
osteosclerosis
    o. congenita
    o. fragilis
    o. myelofibrosis
osteosis
    o. cutis
    o. eburnisans monomelica
    parathyroid o.
osteosynovitis
osteotelangiectasia
osteothrombophlebitis
osteothrombosis
otalgia
    o. dentalis

otalgia *(continued)*
    geniculate o.
    o. intermittens
    reflex o.
    secondary o.
    tabetic o.
otitis
    o. desquamativa
    o. diphtheritica
    o. externa
    o. labyrinthica
    o. mastoidea
    o. media
    mucosis o.
    o. mycotica
    o. sclerotica
otoantritis
otocerebritis
otoconia
otodynia
otoencephalitis
otolithiasis
otomastoiditis
otomucormycosis
Otomyces
    O. hageni
    O. purpureus
otomycosis
    o. aspergillina
otomyiasis
otoneuralgia
otopyorrhea
otorrhagia
otorrhea
    cerebrospinal fluid o.
otosclerosis
ototoxic
Otto disease

Additional Entries

ovalocytosis
ovarialgia
ovarian
   o. cyst
   o. tumor
ovaritis
ovary

ovary *(continued)*
   adenocystic o.
   oyster o's
   polycystic o.
Oxyuris
   O. incognita
   O. vermicularis

Additional Entries

Additional Entries

P

P. (Plasmodium; Proteus)
PA (pernicious anemia; primary amenorrhea; primary anemia)
Paas' disease
pachyacria
pachydermoperiostosis
pachymeningitis
    chronic adhesive p.
    fibrous hypertrophic p.
pachymeningopathy
pachynema
pachyonychia
    p. congenita
pachyperiostitis
pachyperitonitis
pachypleuritis
pachysalpingitis
pachysalpingo-ovaritis
pachyvaginalitis
pachyvaginitis
    cystic p.
Paecilomyces
paecilomycosis
PAFIB (paroxysmal atrial fibrillation)
Paget's disease
PAH (pulmonary artery hypertension)
Pahvant Valley fever
pain
    fulgurant p's
    heterotopic p.
    homotopic p.
    ideogenous p.
    lancinating p.

pain *(continued)*
    phantom limb p.
    referred p.
    terebrating p.
palatitis
palatognathous
pale infarct
palindromia
palmar
    p. fibromatosis
palpitation
palsy
    Bell's p.
    birth p.
    brachial p.
    bulbar p.
    cerebral p.
    crossed leg p.
    diver's p.
    Erb's p.
    facial p.
    ischemic p.
    Klumpke's p.
    Landry's p.
    ocular muscle p.
    progressive bulbar p.
    progressive supranuclear p.
    pseudobulbar p.
    radial p.
    Saturday night p.
    scriveners' p.
    shaking p.
    spastic bulbar p.
    Todd's p.

Additional Entries

palsy *(continued)*
    transverse p.
    wasting p.
Paludina
paludism
PAM (pulmonary alveolar microlithiasis)
PAN (periodic alternating nystagmus)
panacinar emphysema
Pancoast's tumor
pancreas
    aberrant p.
    Baggenstoss change in p.
pancreatic
    p. cholera
    p. tumor
pancreatitis
    calcifying p.
    hemorrhagic p.
    necrotizing p.
    relapsing p.
pancreatolithiasis
pancytopenia
    autoimmune p.
    Fanconi's p.
panencephalitis
    Pette-Doring p.
    subacute sclerosing p.
panhemocytophthisis
panhypopituitarism
    postpubertal p.
    prepubertal p.
panmyelosis
Panner's disease
panniculitis
    mesenteric p.
    metastatic p.

panniculitis *(continued)*
    nodular nonsuppurative p.
    relapsing febrile nodular p.
panophthalmitis
Panstrongylus
PAOD (peripheral arterial occlusive disease)
PAP (primary atypical pneumonia)
papillary
    p. adenocarcinoma
    p. adenoma
    p. adenomatous polyp
    p. carcinoma
    p. cystadenocarcinoma
    p. cystadenoma
    p. cystadenoma lymphomatosum
    p. ependymoma
    p. hidradenoma
    p. hyperplasia
    p. necrosis
    p. serous cystadenocarcinoma
    p. serous cystadenoma
    p. syringadenoma
    p. transitional cell carcinoma
papilledema
papillitis
    anal p.
    chronic lingual p.
    necrotizing p.
    optic p.
papilloma
    basal cell p.
    choroid plexus p.

Additional Entries

papilloma *(continued)*
    cutaneous p.
    fibroepithelial p.
    hirsutoid p's of penis
    Hopmann's p.
    hyperkeratotic p.
    intracystic p.
    intraductal p.
    keratotic p.
    Shope p.
    squamous cell p.
    transitional cell p.
    verrucous p.
    villous p.
papillomatosis
    confluent and reticulate p.
    intraductal p.
papillomatous
papillomavirus
Papillon-Lefevre syndrome
Papovaviridae
papovavirus
pappataci
    p. fever
    p. fever virus
papulonecrotic tuberculid
paracholera
Paracoccidioides
    P. brasiliensis
paracoccidioidomycosis
paracolitis
Paracolobactrum
    P. aerogenoides
    P. arizonae
    P. coliforme
    P. intermedium
paracolon bacilli
paracolpitis

paracoxalgia
paradoxical
    p. embolus
    p. infarct
paraffinoma
Parafossarulus
paraganglioma
    chromaffin p.
    nonchromaffin p.
paragonimiasis
Paragonimus
    P. africanus
    P. caliensis
    P. heterotermus
    P. kellicotti
    P. mexicanus
    P. westermani
Paragordius
    P. cintus
    P. tricuspidatus
    P. varius
paragranuloma
    Hodgkin's p.
parainfluenza virus, Types I-4
parakeratosis
    p. scutularis
paralbuminemia
paralysis
    abducens p.
    p. of accommodation
    acute ascending spinal p.
    acute atrophic p.
    acute bulbar p.
    acute infectious p.
    acute wasting p.
    p. agitans
    alcoholic p.
    ascending p.

Additional Entries

paralysis *(continued)*
- asthenic bulbar p.
- Bell's p.
- birth p.
- brachial p.
- Brown-Sequard's p.
- bulbar p.
- cerebral p.
- Chastek p.
- circumflex p.
- compression p.
- congenital p.
- Dejerine-Klumpke p.
- diphtheric p.
- diver's p.
- Erb's p.
- Erb-Duchenne p.
- familial periodic p.
- infectious bulbar p.
- immunologic p.
- ischemic p.
- Landry's p.
- Millard-Gubler p.
- narcosis p.
- oculomotor p.
- peripheral p.
- Pott's p.
- pressure p.
- progressive bulbar p.
- radial p.
- sensory p.
- spastic spinal p.
- tick p.
- Todd's p.
- trigeminal p.
- vasomotor p.
- Volkmann's p.
- wasting p.

paralysis *(continued)*
- Weber's p.
- Werdnig-Hoffmann p.

Paramecium
- P. coli

parametritis
paramyotonia
- p. congenita

paramyxovirus
paraneoplastic syndrome
paranoid schizophrenia
paraparesis
paraphimosis
paraphyseal cyst
paraplegia
- alcoholic p.
- ataxic p.
- cerebral p.
- Erb's p.
- flaccid p.
- peripheral p.
- Pott's p.
- reflex p.
- senile p.
- spastic p.
- syphilitic p.
- toxic p.

Paraponera
parapraxia
paraproteinemia
parapsoriasis
- p. en plaque
- p. lichenoides et varioliformis acuta

Parasaccharomyces
- P. ashfordi

parasite
- ectozoic p.

Additional Entries

parasite *(continued)*
    entozoic p.
    extracellular p.
    facultative p.
    intermittent p.
    intracellular p.
    malarial p.
    metazoan p.
    obligate p.
    protozoan p.
    spurious p.
parasitemia
parasitic
    p. ectopic pregnancy
    p. embolus
    p. fetus
    p. twin
paratuberculous pneumonia
paratyphoid
    p. A and B
    p. fever
paravirus
parenchymatitis
paresis
paresthesia
Parinaud's syndrome
parkinsonism
Parkinson's
    disease
    facies
Park's aneurysm
paronychia
    herpetic p.
parosteal
    p. osteoma
    p. osteosarcoma
parotiditis
parotitis

parotitis *(continued)*
    infectious p.
paroxysmal
    p. auricular tachycardia
    p. cold hemoglobinuria
    p. dyspnea
    p. myoglobinuria
    p. nocturnal dyspnea
    p. ventricular tachycardia
parrot fever
Parrot's disease
Parry's disease
Paryphostomum
    P. sufrartyfex
PAS (pulmonary artery stenosis)
Pasteurella
    P. haemolytica
    P. multocida
    P. pestis
    P. pneumotropica
    P. pseudotuberculosis
    P. septica
    P. tularensis
    P. ureae
pasteurellosis
PAT (paroxysmal atrial tachycardia)
Patau's syndrome
Paterson-Kelly syndrome
Pautrier microabscess
PBC (primary biliary cirrhosis)
PBN (paralytic brachial neuritis)
PCD (polycystic disease)
PCV (polycythemia vera)
PCV-M (myeloid metaplasia with polycythemia vera)
PD (Parkinson's disease)
Pectobacterium

Additional Entries

Pectobacterium *(continued)*
    P. carotovorum
Pediculoides
    P. ventricosus
pediculosis
Pediculus
    P. humanus capitis
    P. humanus corporis
    P. inguinalis
    P. pubis
Pel-Ebstein fever
Pelger-Huet nuclear anomaly
peliosis
    p. hepatis
Pelizaeus-Merzbacher disease
Pellegrini's disease
pelvic endometriosis
Pemberton's sign
pemphigus
    benign mucous membrane p.
    p. erythematosus
    familial benign p.
    p. foliaceus
    p. neonatorum
    p. vegetans
    p. vulgaris
Pendred's syndrome
penicillinosis
Penicillium
    P. barbae
    P. bouffardi
    P. minimum
    P. montoyai
    P. notatum
    P. patulum
    P. spinulosum
Pentastoma

Pentastoma *(continued)*
    P. constrictum
    P. denticulatum
    P. taenioides
pentastomiasis
Pentatrichomonas
    P. ardin delteili
pentatrichomoniasis
PEO (progressive external ophthalmoplegia)
peptic
    p. esophagitis
    p. ulcer
Peptococcus
    P. anaerobius
    P. asaccharolyticus
    P. constellatus
    P. magnus
    P. prevotti
Peptostreptococcus
    P. anaerobius
    P. intermedius
    P. lanceolatus
    P. micros
    P. productus
perforated
    p. diverticulitis
    p. gastric ulcer
    p. ulcer
perforation
    inflammatory p.
periapical
    p. abscess
    p. granuloma
periappendicitis
periarteritis
    p. gummosa
    p. nodosa

Additional Entries

periarteritis *(continued)*
    syphilitic p.
pericanalicular
    p. fibroadenoma
pericarditis
    adherent p.
    adhesive p.
    bacterial p.
    carcinomatous p.
    constrictive p.
    fibrinous p.
    fungal p.
    hemorrhagic p.
    idiopathic p.
    mediastinal p.
    obliterative p.
    purulent p.
    rheumatic p.
    serofibrinous p.
    suppurative p.
    tuberculous p.
    uremic p.
    viral p.
pericholangitis
periductal mastitis
perihepatitis
perinephric
    p. abscess
perinephritis
perineural
    p. fibroblastoma
periodic
    p. disease
    p. paralysis, familial
periodontitis
perioophoritis
periosteal
    p. fibroma

periosteal *(continued)*
    p. fibrosarcoma
    p. sarcoma
periosteitis
    p. fibrosa
periostitis
periostosis
peripheral
    p. edema
    p. necrosis
    p. neuropathy
    p. odontogenic fibroma
    p. vascular disease
periportal
    p. cardiomyopathy
    p. necrosis
perisplenitis
    hyaline p.
perithelioma
peritonitis
    acute diffuse p.
    fibrinous p.
    gonogoccal p.
    localized p.
    meconium p.
    septic p.
peritonsillar
    p. abscess
perivasculitis
pernicious
    p. anemia
    p. malaria
peroneal muscular atrophy
pertussis
petechia (petechiae)
petechial
    p. hemorrhage
petit mal epilepsy

Additional Entries

petriellidiosis
Petriellidium
    P. boydii
petrositis
petrosooccipital synchondrosis
Peutz-Jeghers syndrome
Peyronie's disease
Pfeiffer's
    bacillus
    disease
    phenomenon
PFT (posterior fossa tumor)
PG (pyoderma gangrenosum)
PH (prostatic hypertrophy; pulmonary hypertension)
phacomalacia
phacomatosis
phacosclerosis
phaeohyphomycosis
phakomatosis
pharyngitis
pharyngoconjunctival fever
pharyngolaryngitis
Phialophora
    P. compactum
    P. dermatitidis
    P. gougerotii
    P. jeanselmei
    P. mutabilis
    P. parasitica
    P. repens
    P. richardsiae
    P. spinifera
    P. verrucosa
phimosis
phlebarteriectasia
phlebectasia
phlebitis
phlebosclerosis
phlebothrombosis
Phlebotomus
    P. argentipes
    P. chinensis
    P. intermedius
    P. macedonicum
    P. noguchi
    P. papatasii
    P. sergenti
    P. verrucarum
    P. vexator
phlebotomus
    p. fever
    p. fever virus
phlegmasia
    p. alba dolens
    p. cerulea dolens
Phlegmonous adenitis
phlyctenulosis
phocomelia
Phoma
    P. hibernica
phosphatemia
phosphatid histiocytosis
photoretinitis
PHP (primary hyperparathyroidism)
phrenoplegia
phthiriasis
Phthirus
    P. pubis
Phycomycetes
phycomycosis
Physaloptera
    P. caucasica
    P. mordens
physalopteriasis
Phytobdella

Additional Entries

PI (pulmonary infarction)
pia-arachnitis
Pick's
    disease
    tubular adenoma
pickwickian disease
picornavirus
PID (pelvic inflammatory disease)
PIE (pulmonary interstitial emphysema)
Piedraia
    P. hortae
Pierre Robbin syndrome
pigeon breast
pigment
    calculous p.
    cirrhosis p.
    melanotic p.
pigmentary
    p. cirrhosis
    p. degeneration
    p. dermatosis
pigmented
    p. pilocytic astrocytoma
    p. purpuric lichenoid dermatitis
    p. villonodular synovitis
    p. villonodular tenosynovitis
piloid astrocytoma
pilomatrixoma
pilonidal
    p. cyst
    p. sinus
pinealoma
pinworm
pipestem cirrhosis

pituitary
    p. dwarfism
    p. endocrine disorder
    p. gonadotrophic failure
    p. myxedema
    p. tumor
pityriasis
    p. alba
    p. capitis
    p. lichenoides et varioliformis acuta
    p. linguae
    p. pilaris
    p. rosea
    p. rubra pilaris
    p. versicolor
Pityrosporon
    P. orbiculare
    P. ovale
    P. versicolor
placentitis
plague
    p. bacillus
    black p.
    bubonic p.
    cellulocutaneous p.
    hemorrhagic p.
    pneumonic p.
    septicemic p.
    sylvatic p.
    urban p.
plantar fibromatosis
plaque
    atheromatous p.
    Hollenhorst p's
    McCallum's p.
    senile p.
plasma

Additional Entries

plasma *(continued)*
   p. dyscrasia
plasmacytic
   p. leukemia
   p. myeloma
plasmacytoma
plasmacytosis
plasmarrhexis
Plasmodium
   P. falciparum
   P. malariae
   P. ovale
   P. pleuodyniae
   P. vivax
   P. vivax minuta
plasmodium
   exoerythrocytic p.
plasmoptysis
platinosis
Platyhelminthes
pleocytosis
pleomorphic
   p. carcinoma
   p. lipoma
Pleospora
Plesiomonas shigelloides
pleural
   p. effusion
   p. fibroma
   p. friction rub
pleuralgia
pleurisy
   fibrinous p.
pleuritis
   acute fibrinous p.
   fibrinous p.
   obliterative p.
pleurodynia

pleurohepatitis
pleuropneumonia
PLEVA (pityriasis lichenoides et varioliformis acuta)
plexiform
   p. neurofibroma
   p. neuroma
plexitis
PLT (psittacosis-lymphogranuloma venereum-trachoma)
Plummer's disease
Plummer-Vinson syndrome
PLV (panleukopenia virus)
PMA (progressive muscular atrophy)
PMC (pseudomembranous colitis)
PMD (primary myocardial disease; progressive muscular dystrophy)
PMF (progressive massive fibrosis)
PML (progressive multifocal leukoencephalopathy)
PN (periarteritis nodosa; peripheral neuropathy; pneumonia; positional nystagmus; pyelonephritis)
PND (paroxysmal nocturnal dyspnea)
pneumarthrosis
pneumatocele
pneumatosis
   p. cystoides intestinalis
   p. intestinalis cystica
pneumobacillus
   Friedlander's p.

Additional Entries

pneumococcal
pneumococcus
Pneumocystis
    P. carinii
pneumocystosis
pneumolithiasis
pneumonia
    acute gelatinous p.
    aspiration p.
    atypical p.
    bronchial p.
    chemical p.
    confluent p.
    desquamative interstitial p.
    diffuse p.
    focal p.
    Friedlander's p.
    fungal p.
    gangrenous p.
    giant cell p.
    Hemophilus influenzae p.
    hemorrhagic p.
    hypostatic p.
    inhalation p.
    interstitial p.
    Klebsiella p.
    lipid p.
    lipoid p.
    lobar p.
    lobular p.
    mycoplasmal p.
    organized p.
    partuberculous p.
    Pittsburgh p. agent
    plasma cell p.
    pneumococcal p.
    primary atypical p.

pneumonia *(continued)*
    primary influenza virus p.
    rheumatic p.
    staphylococcal p.
    streptococcal p.
    tuberculous p.
    unresolved p.
    uremic p.
    viral p.
pneumonic plague
pneumonitis
    acute interstitial p.
    aspiration p.
    desquamative interstitial p.
    granulomatous p.
    interstitial p.
    lymphocytic interstitial p.
    malarial p.
    pneumocystis p.
    rheumatic p.
    uremic p.
pneumonocirrhosis
pneumonomelanosis
pneumonomoniliasis
pneumonomycosis
pneumonophthisis
pneumonopleuritis
pneumothorax
    spontaneous p.
pneumovirus
PNH (paroxysmal nocturnal hemoglobinuria)
poikilocytosis
poikilodermia
    p. atrophicans vasculare Civatte's p.
poikilodermatomyositis

Additional Entries

poisoning
    antimony p.
    arsenic p.
    blood p.
    carbon disulfide p.
    carbon monoxide p.
    chloroform p.
    cyanide p.
    desquamative interstitial p.
    ethyl alcohol p.
    heavy metal p.
    lead p.
    manganese p.
    mercury p.
    methyl alcohol p.
    naphthol p.
    nitroanilene p.
    oxygen p.
    paraldehyde p.
    salmonellal p.
    scombroid p.
    tetrachlorethane p.
    thallium p.
polio
poliodystrophia
    p. cerebri
polioencephalitis
polioencephalomeningomyelitis
polioencephalomyelitis
poliomyelencephalitis
poliomyelitis
    acute anterior p.
    acute lateral p.
    anterior p.
    ascending p.
    bulbar p.
    cerebral p.

poliomyelitis *(continued)*
    endemic p.
    immunization reaction p.
    spinal paralytic p.
    virus p.
poliomyeloencephalitis
poliovirus, types I, II, III
polyangiitis
polyarteritis nodosa
polyarthritis
polychromasia
polychromatocytosis
polychromatosis
polychondritis
    chronic atrophic p.
    relapsing p.
polycystic
    p. change
    p. kidney
    p. ovary
    p. ovary syndrome
polycythemia
    p. hypertonica
    myelopathic p.
    p. rubra
    splenomegalic p.
    p. versa
polycytosis
polydactyly
polyemia
    p. aquosa
    p. hyperalbuminosa
    p. polycythaemica
    p. serosa
polyendocrine adenomatosis
polyhydramnios
polymastia
polymyalgia rheumatica

Additional Entries

polymyositis
polyneuritic-type hypertrophic
　　muscular atrophy
polyneuritis
polyneuropathy
polyostotic fibrous dysplasia
polyp
　　adenomatous p.
　　aural p.
　　cardiac p.
　　cervical p.
　　choanal p.
　　cockscomb p.
　　colorectal p.
　　endometrial p.
　　fibroepithelial p.
　　gastric p.
　　granulomatous p.
　　Hopmann's p.
　　hydatid p.
　　inflammatory p.
　　laryngeal p.
　　lymphoid p.
　　nasal p.
　　papillary adenomatous p.
　　placental p.
　　retention p.
　　umbilical p.
polyparasitism
polyphagia
polypoid
　　p. adenoma
　　p. hyperplasia
polyposis
　　p. coli
　　familial p.
　　familial intestinal p.
　　p. gastrica

polyradiculoneuritis
polyserositis
polysyndactyly
polysynovitis
polytendinitis
polytendinobursitis
polytenosynovitis
Pompe's disease
Poncet's disease
Pontiac fever
poorly differentiated
　　lymphocytic lymphoma
Porocephalus
　　P. armillatus
　　P. clavatus
　　P. constrictus
　　P. denticulatus
porokeratosis
　　Mibelli's p.
porphyria
　　acute intermittent p.
　　congenital p.
　　p. cutanea tarda
　　p. erythropoietica
　　hepatic p.
　　latent p.
　　photosensitive p.
porta hepatis
portal
　　p. cirrhosis
　　p. hypertension
Posada-Wernicke disease
posthemorrhagic anemia
posthepatic cirrhosis
postinfectious
　　p. encephalomyelitis
　　p. glomerulonephritis
postnecrotic cirrhosis

Additional Entries

postpubertal
    p. hyperpituitarism
    p. panhypopituitarism
posttransfusion hepatitis
Pott's aneurysm
Powassan virus
poxvirus
Prader-Willi syndrome
precancerous dysplasia
Preiser's disease
Preisz-Nocard bacillus
preleukemia
presenile dementia
primary
    p. adrenal insufficiency
    p. amenorrhea
Prinzmetal's angina
proctatresia
proctitis
proctocele
proctoptosis
progonoma
    melanotic p.
progranulocytic leukemia
progressive
    p. bulbar palsy
    p. cerebellar dyssynergia
    p. massive fibrosis
    p. multifocal
        leukoencephalopathy
    p. muscular dystrophy
    p. pigmentary dermatosis
    p. spinal muscular atrophy
    p. systemic sclerosis
proliferative
    p. chronic arthritis
    p. endometrium
    p. glomerulonephritis

proliferative *(continued)*
    p. inflammation
    p. myositis
    p. synovitis
propagating thrombosis
Propionibacterium
    P. acnes
    P. avidum
    P. granulosum
    P. lymphophilum
prosopagnosia
prosopalgia
prosoplasia
prostatic tumor
prostatitis
prostatocystitis
prostration
    heat p.
proteinemia
proteinosis
    alveolar p.
    lipoid p.
proteinuria
    Bence-Jones p.
Proteus
    P. inconstans
    P. mirabilis
    P. morganii
    P. OX-K, OX-2, OX-19
    P. rettgeri
    P. stuartii
    P. vulgaris
Protodiastolic gallop
protoplasmic astrocytoma
Prototheca
    P. ciferrii
    P. filamenta
    P. portoricensin

Additional Entries

Protheca *(continued)*
    P. segbwema
    P. wickerhamii
    P. zopfi
prurigo nodularis
pruritis
    p. ani
    p. vulvae
PS (pulmonary stenosis)
psammomatous meningioma
pseudarthrosis
pseudobulbar palsy
pseudocholesteatoma
pseudochromhidrosis
pseudocirrhosis
pseudodiverticulum
pseudolymphoma
pseudomelanosis coli
pseudomembranous
    p. acute inflammation
    p. colitis
    p. enterocolitis
Pseudomonas
    P. acidovorans
    P. aeruginosa
    P. alcaligenes
    P. cepacia
    P. diminuta
    P. eisenbergii
    P. fluorescens
    P. fragi
    P. kingii
    P. mallei
    P. maltophilia
    P. multivorans
    P. nonliquefaciens
    P. paucimobilis
    P. pseudoalcaligenes

Pseudomonas *(continued)*
    P. pseudomallei
    P. putida
    P. putrefaciens
    P. pyocyanea
    P. stutzeri
    P. syncyanea
    P. testosteroni
    P. viscosa
Pseudomonilia
pseudomucinous
    p. cystadenocarcinoma
    p. cystadenoma
    p. degeneration
pseudomyiasis
pseudomyxoma peritonei
pseudoneurotic schizophrenia
pseudoparakeratosis
pseudopolycythemia
pseudopolyposis
pseudopseudohypoparathyroidism
pseudosarcoma
pseudosarcomatous fasciitis
pseudosclerosis
    Jakob-Creutzfeldt p.
    Westphal-Strumpell p.
pseudoxanthoma elasticum
PSGN (poststreptococcal
    glomerulonephritis)
psittacosis
psoas abscess
psoriasiform dermatitis
psoriasis
    exfoliative p.
    pustular p.
    p. vulgaris
PSP (progressive supranuclear
    palsy)

Additional Entries

psychomotor epilepsy
PT (paroxysmal tachycardia)
PTA (persistent truncus arteriosus)
PTE (pulmonary thromboembolism)
PTED (pulmonary thromboembolic disease)
pterygium
    p. coli
    congenital p.
PTI (persistent tolerant infection)
ptosis
ptyalism
PU (peptic ulcer)
PUD (pulmonary disease)
PUE (pyrexia of unknown etiology)
Pullularia
    P. pullulans
pulmonary
    p. adenomatosis
    p. alveolar microlithiasis
    p. congestion
    p. distomiasis
    p. edema
    p. embolism
    p. emphysema
    p. fibrosis
    p. hemosiderosis
    p. hypertension
    p. infarct
    p. interstitial emphysema
    p. osteoarthropathy
    p. pneumonitis
    p. sarcoidosis
pulpitis

pulpitis *(continued)*
    putrescent p.
PUO (pyrexia of unknown origin)
pure red cell aplasia
purpura
    allergic p.
    anaphylactoid p.
    p. annularis telangiectodes
    fibrinolytic p.
    Henoch's p.
    Schonlein's p.
    thrombocytopenic p.
    thrombotic thrombocytopenic p.
purulent
pus
    p. bonum et laudabile
    ichorous p.
    sanious p.
pustular
    p. psoriasis
putrescent pulpitis
PV (polycythemia vera)
PVC (premature ventricular contraction; pulmonary venous congestion)
PVD (peripheral vascular disease)
PVS (premature ventricular systole)
PVT (paroxysmal ventricular tachycardia; portal vein thrombosis)
Px (pneumothorax)
PXE (pseudoxanthoma elasticum)
pyelitis

Additional Entries

pyelitis *(continued)*
    p. cystica
    p. glandularis
pyelonephritis
pyknodysostosis
pyknosis
pylephlebitis
pyloric stenosis
pyoderma gangrenosum
pyonephrosis

pyorrhea
    p. alveolaris
    Schmutz p.
pyostomatitis
    p. vegetans
Pyrenochaeta
    P. romeroi
pyrexia
    Pel-Ebstein p.
pyuria

Additional Entries

Additional Entries

Q

Quain's degeneration
Queckenstedt's sign
Quenu-Muret sign
Quervain's disease

Queyrat's erythroplasia
Quincke's disease
Quinquaud's disease

Additional Entries

Additional Entries

R

R. (Rickettsia)
RA (rheumatoid arthritis)
rabies virus
racemose aneurysm
rachischisis
rachitis
radiculitis
radiculoganglionitis
radiculomeningomyelitis
radiculomyelopathy
radiculoneuropathy
radiculopathy
radiodermatitis
Raeder's paratrigeminal syndrome
RAH (right atrial hypertrophy)
Raillietina
    R. celebensis
    R. demerariensis
Ramsay Hunt syndrome
Ranikhet disease
RAS (renal artery stenosis)
Rasmussen's aneurysm
rat bite fever
Rathke's pouch tumor
Rayer's disease
Raymond-Cestan syndrome
Raynaud's disease
RBBB (right bundle branch block)
RCS (reticulum cell sarcoma)
RD (Raynaud's disease)
RDS (respiratory distress syndrome)
rectocele
Recklinghausen-Applebaum disease
Recklinghausen's disease
Recklinghausen's disease of bone
Reclus' disease
Reed-Hodgkin disease
Refetoff syndrome
reflux
    gastroesophageal r.
    hepatojugular r.
    vesicoureteral r.
Refsum's disease
regional
    r. colitis
    r. enteritis
    r. enterocolitis
    r. ileitis
regurgitation
    cardiac valvular r.
Reichmann's disease
Reifenstein's syndrome
Reiter's syndrome
relapsing fever
renal
    r. adenoma
    r. amyloidosis
    r. calculi
    r. cell carcinoma
    r. cortical necrosis
    r. dysplasia
    r. edema
    r. failure
    r. glycosuria
    r. hypertension
    r. infarct

Additional Entries

renal *(continued)*
    r. osteodystrophy
    r. rickets
    r. stones
    r. tubular acidosis
    r. vein thrombosis
Rendu-Osler disease
Rendu-Osler-Weber disease
Renpenning's syndrome
reparative giant cell granuloma
reserve
    r. cell carcinoma
    r. cell hyperplasia
respiration
    Cheyne-Stokes r.
    cogwheel r.
    interrupted r.
    Kussmaul r.
respiratory
    r. acidosis
    r. alkalosis
    r. disorder
    r. distress syndrome
    r. exanthematous virus
    r. failure
    r. rate disorder
    r. rhythm disorder
    r. syncytial virus
    r. syndrome
retention
    r. cyst
    r. polyp
    urinary r.
reticulocytopenia
reticulocytosis
reticuloendothelial
    r. cell hyperplasia
    r. sarcoma
reticuloendotheliosis
    systemic r.
reticulohistiocytic granuloma
reticulohistiocytoma
reticulosis
    medullary histiocytic r.
reticulum cell
    r. c. hyperplasia
    r. c. lymphosarcoma
    r. c. sarcoma
retinal
    r. anlage tumor
    r. detachment
    r. microaneurysm
retinitis
    r. pigmentosa
    r. proliferans
retinopathy
    diabetic r.
Retortamonas
    R. intestinalis
retrolental fibroplasia
retroperitoneal fibromatosis
retroperitonitis
retrovirus
Rettgerella rettgeri
Reye's syndrome
RF (rheumatic fever)
Rhabditis
    R. hominis
Rhabdomonas
rhabdomyoma
rhabdomyosarcoma
    alveolar r.
    embryonal r.
rhabdovirus
RHD (rheumatic heart disease)
rheumatic

Additional Entries

rheumatic *(continued)*
    r. arteritis
    r. arthralgia
    r. endocarditis
    r. fever
    r. heart disease
    r. myocarditis
    r. pneumonia
    r. valvulitis
rheumatism
rheumatoid
    r. ankylosing spondylitis
    r. aortitis
    r. arteritis
    r. arthritis
    r. episcleritis
    r. heart disease
    r. scleritis
rhinitis
    allergic r.
    atrophic r.
    fetid r.
    r. sicca
    vasomotor r.
Rhinocladium
rhinocleisis
rhinoentomophthoromycosis
rhinonasopharyngitis
rhinophycomycosis
rhinophyma
rhinorrhea
rhinoscleroma
rhinosporidiosis
Rhinosporidium seeberi
rhinovirus
Rh immunization syndrome
Rhizoglyphus
    R. parasiticus

Rhizopus
    R. niger
    R. nigricans
    R. rhizopodoformis
Rhodesian trypanosomiasis
Rhodophyllus sinuatus
Rhodotorula
    R. mucilaginosa
    R. rubra
rhodotorulosis
rhopheocytosis
RI (regional ileitis; respiratory illness)
Ribas-Torres disease
riboflavin deficiency
Richards-Rundle syndrome
Richet's aneurysm
Richter's syndrome
Rickettsia
    R. akamushi
    R. akari
    R. australis
    R. burnetii
    R. canada
    R. conorii
    R. diaporica
    R. mooseri
    R. muricola
    R. nipponica
    R. orientalis
    R. pavlovskii
    R. pediculi
    R. prowazekii
    R. quintana
    R. rickettsii
    R. sibiricus
    R. tsutsugamushi
    R. typhi

Additional Entries

Rickettsia *(continued)*
    R. wolhynica
rickettsia
Rickettsiaceae
rickettsialpox
Riedel's thyroiditis
Rieger's syndrome
Riehl's melanosis
Rift Valley fever
Rift Valley fever virus
Riga-Fede disease
Riga's disease
Riggs' disease
rigor mortis
Riley-Day syndrome
Riley-Smith syndrome
ringworm
Ritter's disease
RMSF (Rocky Mountain spotted fever)
Roaf's syndrome
Robert's syndrome
Robinow's syndrome
Robinson's disease
Robin's syndrome
Robles' disease
Rocky Mountain spotted fever
Rodrigues' aneurysm
Roger
    maladie de R.
rolandic epilepsy
Roger's disease
Rokitansky-Kuster-Hauser syndrome
Rokitansky's disease
Romana sign
Romano-Ward syndrome
Romberg's disease

Rose disease
Rosenbach's syndrome
Rosenthal-Kloepfer syndrome
Rosenthal's syndrome
roseola
    r. infantum
    r. infantum virus
Rosewater's syndrome
Rossbach's disease
Rot-Bernhardt disease
Rothmann-Makai syndrome
Rothmund-Thompson syndrome
Roth's disease
Rotor's syndrome
Rot's disease
Rotter's syndrome
Rougnon-Heberden disease
roundworm
Rous sarcoma virus
Roussy-Dejerine syndrome
Roussy-Levy's disease
Rovsing syndrome
RPGN (rapidly progressive glomerulonephritis)
RSA (reticulum cell sarcoma)
RSV (Rous sarcoma virus)
Rubarth's disease
rubella virus
rubeola virus
Rubinstein's syndrome
Rubinstein-Taybi syndrome
rudimentary testis syndrome
Rud's syndrome
Rummo's disease
runt disease
ruptured
    r. aneurysm
    r. ectopic pregnancy

Additional Entries

ruptured *(continued)*
    r. myocardial infarct
RURTI (recurrent upper respiratory tract infection)
Rusconi's anus
Russell-Silver syndrome
Russell's syndrome
Russian spring-summer encephalitis virus
Rust's disease
Ruysch's disease
RV (rubella virus)
RVT (renal vein thrombosis)

Additional Entries

Additional Entries

S

S. (Salmonella; Schistosoma; Spirillum; Staphylococcus; Streptococcus)
SA (sarcoma)
SAB (significant asymptomatic bacteriuria)
Sabin-Feldman syndrome
Saccharomyces
    S. albicans
    S. anginae
    S. apiculatus
    S. cantliei
    S. capillitii
    S. carlsbergensis
    S. cerevisiae
    S. soprogenus
    S. epidermica
    S. galacticolus
    S. glutinis
    S. hominis
    S. lemonnieri
    S. mellis
    S. mycoderma
    S. neoformans
    S. pastorianus
saccharomycosis
saccular
    s. aneurysm
    s. bronchiectasis
Sachs' disease
Saethre-Chotzen syndrome
SAH (subarachnoid hemorrhage)
St. Agatha's disease
St. Aignon's disease
St. Anthony's disease
St. Appolonia's disease
St. Avertin's disease
St. Avidus' disease
St. Blasius' disease
St. Dymphna's disease
St. Erasmus' disease
St. Fiacre's disease
St. Gervasius' disease
St. Gotthard's tunnel disease
St. Hubert's disease
St. Job's disease
St. Louis encephalitis
St. Louis encephalitis virus
St. Mathurin's disease
St. Modestus' disease
St. Roch's disease
St. Sement's disease
St. Valentine's disease
St. Zachary's disease
Salisbury common cold virus
salivary virus
Salmonella
    S. arizonae
    S. choleraesuis
    S. derby
    S. enteritidis
    S. gallinarum
    S. hirschfeldii
    S. indiana
    S. minnesota
    S. montevideo
    S. muenchen
    S. newington
    S. oranienburg
    S. paratyphi, A, B, C

Additional Entries

Salmonella *(continued)*
    S. schottmulleri
    S. sendai
    S. thompson
    S. typhi
    S. typhimurium
    S. typhisuis
    S. typhosa
    S. virginia
salmonellosis
salpingitis
    follicular s.
    s. isthmica nodosa
salpingocele
salpingolithiasis
salpingo-oophoritis
salpingoperitonitis
Sanarelli-Shwartzman phenomenon
Sanchez Salorio syndrome
Sanders' disease
Sandhoff's disease
Sanfilippo's syndrome
San Joaquin fever
Sarcocystis
sarcoidosis
    s. cordis
    muscular s.
sarcoma
    Abernethy's s.
    adipose s.
    alveolar s.
    ameloblastic s.
    botryoid s.
    s. botryoides
    cerebellar s.
    endometrial stromal s.
    endothelial s.

sarcoma *(continued)*
    Ewing's s.
    giant cell s.
    hemangioendothelial s.
    Hodgkin's s.
    immunoblastic s. of T cells
    Jensen's s.
    Kaposi's s.
    Kupffer cell s.
    leukocytic s.
    lymphangioendothelial s.
    lymphatic s.
    mast cell s.
    meningeal s.
    mesothelial s.
    mixed cell s.
    multiple hemorrhagic s.
    neurogenic s.
    osteogenic s.
    periosteal s.
    reticuloendothelial s.
    reticulum cell s.
    small cell s.
    spindle cell s.
    stromal s.
    synovial s.
    telangiectatic s.
    undifferentiated s.
sarcomatosis
    s. cutis
    general s.
    meningeal s.
Sarcophaga
    S. carnaria
    S. dux
    S. fuscicauda
    S. haemorrhoidalis
    S. nificornis

Additional Entries

Sarcophaga *(continued)*
   S. rubicornis
Sarcoptes
   S. scabiei
sarcoptidosis
sarcosporidiosis
SAS (supravalvular aortic stenosis)
satellitosis
satyriasis
Saunders' disease
Savill's disease
scalded skin syndrome
scalenus anticus syndrome
scarlatina
   s. anginosa
   s. haemorrhagica
   puerperal s.
scarlet fever
SCC (squamous cell carcinoma)
Schafer's syndrome
Schamberg's disease
Schanz's disease
Schaumann's disease
Scheie's syndrome
Schenck's disease
Scheuermann's disease
Schilder's disease
Schilling-type monocytic leukemia
Schimmelbusch's disease
Schirmer's syndrome
Schistosoma
   S. haematobium
   S. intercalatum
   S. japonicum
   S. mansoni
schistosomiasis

schistosomiasis *(continued)*
   cutaneous s.
   eastern s.
   s. haematobia
   hepatic s.
   s. intercalatum
   intestinal s.
   s. japonica
   Manson's s.
   Oriental s.
   pulmonary s.
   urinary s.
   visceral s.
schizophrenia
   acute undifferentiated s.
   catatonic s.
   chronic undifferentiated s.
   hebephrenic s.
   paranoid s.
   pseudoneurotic s.
   schizoaffective s.
   simple s.
Schizophyllum commune
Schizosaccharomyces
Schlatter-Osgood disease
Schlatter's disease
Schmid-Fraccaro syndrome
Schmidt's syndrome
Schmitz's bacillus
Schmorl's
   bacillus
   disease
Schloz's disease
Schonlein-Henoch disease
Schonlein's purpura
Schottmuller's disease
Schridde's disease
Schroeder's disease

Additional Entries

Schuller-Christian disease
Schuller's disease
Schultz syndrome
Schultz's disease
schwannoma
    malignant s.
Schwartz syndrome
Schwediauer's disease
Schweninger-Buzzi disease
scirrhous carcinoma
scleredema
    s. adultorum
sclerema
    s. neonatorum
sclerosing
    s. adenosis
    s. hemangioma
    s. osteitis
    s. sinusitis
sclerosis
    amyotrophic s.
    disseminated s.
    endocardial s.
    endomyocardial s.
    lobar s.
    multiple s.
    primary endocardial s.
    progressive systemic s.
    subacute combined s.
    tuberous s.
scoliosis
Scopulariopsis
    S. americana
    S. aureus
    S. blochi
    S. brevicaulis
    S. cinereus
    S. koningi

Scopulariopsis *(continued)*
    S. minimus
scopulariopsosis
scotoma
scrub typhus
SD (septal defect)
sebaceous
    s. adenocarcinoma
    s. adenoma
    s. carcinoma
    s. cyst
seborrhea
seborrheic
    s. dermatitis
    s. keratosis
Seckel's syndrome
secondary
    s. amenorrhea
    s. constriction
second degree
    s. d. burn
    s. d. frostbite
    s. d. heart block
    s. d. radiation injury
Seitelberger's disease
Selter's disease
Selye syndrome
Semliki Forest virus
Sendai virus
Senear-Usher disease
senile
    s. amyloidosis
    s. atrophy
    s. dementia
    s. elastosis
    s. endometrium
    s. keratosis
    s. plaque

Additional Entries

senility
sensation
    burning s.
    prickling s.
    tingling s.
sepsis
septal
    s. fibrosis of liver
    s. hypertrophy
septal defect
    atrial s. d.
    interatrial s. d.
    interventricular s. d.
    ventricular s. d.
septic
    s. embolus
    s. infarct
    s. shock
septicemia
    bronchopulmonary s.
septicopyemia
septimetritis
septineuritis
sequelae
serofibrinous effusion
serous
    s. acute inflammation
    s. acute synovitis
    s. atrophy
    s. cyst
    s. cystadenocarcinoma, papillary
    s. cystadenoma, papillary
    s. cystoma
    s. effusion
    s. inflammation
Serratia
    S. indica

Serratia *(continued)*
    S. kiliensis
    S. liquefaciens
    S. marcescens
    S. piscatorum
    S. plymuthica
    S. rubidaea
Sertoli-Leydig cell tumor
serum hepatitis
serum hepatitis virus
Sever's disease
Sezary
    reticulosis
    syndrome
SF (scarlet fever)
SH (serum hepatitis)
Shaver's disease
Sheehan's syndrome
Shichito disease
Shiga's bacillus
Shigella
    S. alkalescens
    S. ambigua
    S. arabinotarda Type A, B
    S. boydii
    S. ceylonensis
    S. dispar
    S. dysenteriae
    S. etousae
    S. flexneri
    S. madampensis
    S. newcastle
    S. paradysenteriae
    S. parashigae
    S. schmitzii
    S. shigae
    S. sonnei
    S. wakefield

Additional Entries

shigellosis
shingles
SHO (secondary hypertrophic osteoarthropathy)
shock
    anaphylactic s.
    cardiogenic s.
    colloid s.
    endotoxic s.
    faradic s.
    hemoclastic s.
    hemorrhagic s.
    histamine s.
    hypolycemic s.
    hypovolemic s.
    insulin s.
    micro s.
    neurogenic s.
    osmotic s.
    protein s.
    septic s.
    serum s.
    thyrotoxin s.
    toxic s.
    vasogenic s.
Shope papilloma
Shwachman-Diamond syndrome
Shy-Drager syndrome
sialadenitis
sialolithiasis
sialorrhea
Sicard's syndrome
sicca syndrome
sickle cell
    s. c. anemia
    s. c. disease
    s. c. thalassemia
    s. c. trait

SID (sudden infant death)
sideroachrestic anemia
Siderobacter
sideroblastic anemia
Siderococcus
siderofibrosis
sideropenia
sideropenic dysphagia
sidcrosilicosis
siderosis
SIDS (sudden infant death syndrome)
sigmoiditis
sign
    Babinski's s.
    Blumberg's s.
    Brudzinski's s.
    Chaddock's s.
    Chvostek's s.
    Cullen's s.
    Goodell's s.
    Hegar's s.
    Kernig's s.
    Nikolsky's s.
    Pemberton's s.
    Romana's s.
    Trousseau's s.
    Unschuld's s.
signet ring
    s. r. adenocarcinoma
    s. r. carcinoma
silicosis
Silverskiold's syndrome
Silver's syndrome
Silvestrini-Corda syndrome
Simbu virus
simian sarcoma virus
Simmonds' disease

Additional Entries

Simons' disease
Sindbis virus
sinistrocardia
    isolated s.
sinoatrial
    s. block
sinus
    s. bradycardia
    s. histiocytosis
    inflammatory s.
    s. tract, inflammatory
sinusitis
    sclerosing s.
Siphunculina
Sipple's syndrome
sirenomelia
Sisyrosea
Sjogren-Larsson syndrome
Sjogren's syndrome
skeletal dysplasia
SLE (systemic lupus erythematosus; St. Louis encephalitis)
sleep
    s. apnea
    s. deprivation
sleeping sickness
SLEV (St. Louis encephalitis virus)
SLKC (superior limbic keratoconjunctivitis)
SLR (Streptococcus lactis R)
Sly disease
SM (systolic murmur)
small cell
    s. c. carcinoma
    s. c. sarcoma
smallpox

smallpox *(continued)*
    coherent s.
    confluent s.
    discrete s.
    hemorrhagic s.
    inoculation s.
    malignant s.
    modified s.
    s. virus
Smith-Strang disease
SMON (subacute myelo-optical neuropathy)
soft chancre
SOL (space-occupying lesion)
solar keratosis
solid
    s. carcinoma
    s. teratoma
solitary
    s. cyst
    s. lymphoid nodule
    s. plasmacytoma
SOM (secretory otitis media; serous otitis media)
somasthenia
somatostatinoma
somesthesia
Sonne-Duval bacillus
Sonne dysentery
Sotos' syndrome
South American blastomycosis
sparganosis
Sparganum proliferum
spasm
    torsion s.
spastic
    s. bulbar palsy
    s. colitis

Additional Entries

spastic *(continued)*
    s. gait
spermatocele
spermatogenic
    s. arrest
    s. granuloma
SPH (secondary pulmonary hemosiderosis)
sphaceloderma
Sphaerophorus
    S. necrophorus
spheno-occipital synchondrosis
sphenopetrosal synchondrosis
spherocytosis
    hereditary s.
spheroma
spherophakia
sphincteralgia
sphincterismus
sphincteritis
sphingolipidosis
sphingolipodystrophy
spiradenoma
    cylindromatous s.
    eccrine s.
Spirochaeta
spirochete
    Dutton's s.
spirochetemia
spirochetosis
    s. arthritica
    bronchopulmonary s.
Spirometra
    S. erinaceieuropaei
    S. mansonoides
splanchnectopia
splanchnocele
splanchnodiastasis
splanchnolith
splanchnomegaly
splanchnopathy
splanchnoptosis
splanchnosclerosis
splayfoot
splenadenoma
splenalgia
splenatrophy
splenectopia
splenelcosis
splenemia
splenemphraxis
splenicterus
splenitis
splenocele
splenoceratosis
splenocleisis
splenodynia
splenohepatomegaly
splenokeratosis
splenoma
splenomalacia
splenomegaly
    congestive s.
    Egyptian s.
    Gaucher's s.
    hemolytic s.
    infective s.
    myelophthisis s.
    siderotic s.
    spodogenous s.
    thrombophlebitic s.
    tropical s.
splenomyelomalacia
splenonephroptosis
splenoparectasis
splenopathy

Additional Entries

splenopneumonia
splenoptosis
splenorrhagia
splenosis
spondyalgia
spondylarthritis
    s. ankylopoietica
spondylarthrocace
spondyloarthropathy
spondylexarthrosis
spondylitis
    ankylosing s.
    Bekhterev's s.
    hypertrophic s.
    s. infectiosa
    Kummell's s.
    Marie-Strumpell s.
    muscular s.
    post-traumatic s.
    rheumatoid s.
    rhizomelic s.
    tuberculous s.
    s. typhosa
spondylizema
spondylolisthesis
spondylomalacia
    s. traumatica
spondylopathy
    traumatic s.
spondylopyosis
spondyloschisis
spondylosis
    cervical s.
    s. chronica ankylopoietica
    lumbar s.
    s. uncovertebralis
spongiitis
spongioblastoma

spongioblastoma *(continued)*
    s. multiforme
    s. unipolare
spongiosis
spongiositis
spongy
    s. degenerative-type leukodystrophy
    s. nevus
spontaneous
    s. abortion
    s. pneumothorax
spore
    bacterial s.
    fungal s.
Sporothrix
    S. schenckii
sporotrichosis
Sporotrichum
    S. beurmanni
    S. schenckii
spotted fever
    Rocky Mountain s. f.
Sprinz Nelson syndrome
squamous
    s. metaplasia
    s. papilloma
squamous cell
    s. c. carcinoma
    s. c. carcinoma and adenocarcinoma, mixed
    s. c. carcinoma-in-situ
    s. c. papilloma
SS (Salmonella-Shigella; subaortic stenosis)
SSP (subacute sclerosing panencephalitis)

Additional Entries

stachybotryotoxicosis
Staph (Staphylococcus)
staph (staphylococcus)
staphylococcal
    s. colitis
    s. enteritis
    s. folliculitis
    s. pharyngitis
    s. pneumonia
    s. sinusitis
    s. tonsillitis
staphylococcemia
Staphylococcus
    S. albus
    S. aureus
    S. citreus
    S. epidermidis
    S. pyogenes aureus
    S. pyogenes var. albus
    S. saprophyticus
staphyloma
stasis
    bile s.
    dermatitis s.
    ulcer s.
status
    s. asthmaticus
    s. epilepticus
    s. marmoratus
    s. spongiosis
    s. thymicolymphaticus
STC (soft tissue calcification)
STD (sexually transmitted disease)
steatomatosis
steatopygia
steatorrhea
steatosis

Steinert's disease
Stein-Leventhal syndrome
Stelangium
stem cell
    s. c. leukemia
    s. c. lymphoma
stenosis
    aortic s.
    calcific s.
    caroticovertebral s.
    congenital s.
    hypertrophic pyloric s.
    s. and incompetency
    mitral s.
    nodular calcific s.
    nodular calcific aortic s.
    pyloric s.
    subaortic s.
    valvular s.
stercoraceous ulcer
sternal synchondrosis
Stevens-Johnson syndrome
Stewart-Treves syndrome
stillbirth
    macerated s.
Still's disease
Stokes-Adams syndrome
stomach
    bilocular s.
    dumping s.
    hourglass s.
    sclerotic s.
    thoracic s.
    trifid s.
stomachalgia
stomachodynia
stomal ulcer
stomatalgia

Additional Entries

stomatitis
    allergic s.
    angular s.
    aphthobullous s.
    s. aphthosa
    s. arsenicalis
    bismuth s.
    catarrhal s.
    contact s.
    denture s.
    epidemic s.
    erythematopultaceous s.
    s. exanthematica
    fusospirochetal s.
    gangrenous s.
    gonococcal s.
    gonorrheal s.
    herpetic s.
    infectious s.
    s. intertropica
    lead s.
    s. medicamentosa
    membranous s.
    mercurial s.
    mycotic s.
    s. nicotina
    nonspecific s.
    recurrent aphthous s.
    s. scarlatina
    s. scorbutica
    syphilitic s.
    tropical s.
    ulcerative s.
    uremic s.
    s. venenata
    vesicular s.
    Vincent's s.
stomatocace
stomatocytosis
stamatodynia
stomatodysodia
stomatoglossitis
stomatomalacia
stomatomenia
stomatomycosis
stomatopathy
stomatorrhagia
    s. gingivarum
stomatoschisis
stomoschisis
Stomoxys
    S. calcitrans
stool
    acholic s.
    bilious s.
    caddy s.
    fatty s.
    lienteric s.
    mucous s.
    pea soup s.
    pipe-stem s.
    ribbon s.
    rice-water s's
    sago-grain s.
    silver s.
    tarry s.
storage disease
strabismus
    absolute s.
    accommodative s.
    alternating s.
    concomitant s.
    convergent s.
    cyclis s.
    s. deorsum vergens
    divergent s.

Additional Entries

strabismus *(continued)*
    incomitant s.
    intermittent s.
    internal s.
    kinetic s.
    latent s.
    manifest s.
    mechanical s.
    monocular s.
    muscular s.
    noncomitant s.
    nonparalytic s.
    paralytic s.
    s. sursum vergens
    unilateral s.
    vertical s.
Strachan's syndrome
strangulated hernia
Strengeria
strep (streptococcus)
Streptobacillus
    S. moniliformis
    S. pseudotuberculosis
streptococcal
    s. cellulitis
    s. erysipelas
    s. lymphangitis
    s. nasopharyngitis
    s. pharyngitis
    s. tonsillitis
Streptococceae
Streptococcus
    S. agalactiae
    S. anaerobius
    S. anginosus-constellatus
    S. bovis
    S. cremoris
    S. durans

Streptococcus *(continued)*
    S. equi
    S. equisimilis
    S. evolutus
    S. faecalis
    S. faecium
    S. hemolyticus
    S. intermedius
    S. lactis
    S. liquefaciens
    S. MG
    S. MG-intermedius
    S. microaerophilic
    S. milleri
    S. mitis
    S. mutans
    S. pneumoniae
    S. pyogenes
    S. salivarius
    S. sanguis
    S. uberis
    S. viridans
    S. zooepidemicus
    S. zymogenes
streptococcus
    alpha s.
    anhemolytic s.
    Bargen's s.
    beta s.
    Fehleisen's s.
    gamma s.
    group A s.
    group D s.
    group N s.
    hemolytic s.
    s. MG
    nonhemolytic s.
    s. of Ostertag

Additional Entries

Streptomyces
   S. madurae
   S. pelletieri
   S. somaliensis
streptomycosis
streptotrichosis
striatonigral degeneration
stroke
   apoplectic s.
   heat s.
   lightning s.
   paralytic s.
stromal
   s. endometriosis
   s. hyperplasia
   s. sarcoma
stromatosis
   endometrial s.
Strong's bacillus
Strongyloides
   S. fulleborni
   S. stercoralis
strongyloidiasis
struma
   s. aberranta
   s. calculosa
   s. colloides
   s. endothoracica
   s. fibrosa
   s. follicularis
   Hashimoto's s.
   s. lymphomatosa
   s. maligna
   s. nodosa
   s. ovarii
   s. parenchymatosa
   Riedel's s.
   thymus s.

struma *(continued)*
   s. vasculosa
strumitis
Strumpell's disease
Strumpell-Leichtenstern disease
Strumpell-Lorrain disease
Strumpell-Marie disease
Strumpell-Westphal
   pseudosclerosis
Strunsky's sign
Sturge's disease
Sturge-Weber syndrome
Sturge-Weber-Kalischer
   syndrome
stuttering
   labiochoreic s.
   urinary s.
STVA (subtotal villose atrophy)
stymatosis
subacute
   s. bacterial endocarditis
   s. combined degeneration
   s. combined sclerosis
   s. glomerulonephritis
   s. inflammation
   s. necrotizing
     encephalopathy
   s. sclerosing
     panencephalitis
   s. spongiform
     encephalopathy
subaortic stenosis
   discrete s. s.
   idiopathic hypertrophic s.
     s.
subcutaneous
   s. emphysema
subdural

Additional Entries

subdural *(continued)*
    s. empyema
    s. hematoma
    s. hygroma
subependymal
    s. glioma
subependymoma
subepidermal
    s. fibrosis
subglossitis
subleukemic leukemia
subluxation
    s. of lens
    Volkmann's s.
SUD (sudden unexplained death)
sudanophilic
    s. leukodystrophy
sudden
    s. cardiac death
    s. coronary death
    s. infant death syndrome
Sudeck's atrophy
Sudeck-Leriche syndrome
SUID (sudden unexplained infant death)
sulfatide lipidosis
suppuration
    alveodental s.
suppurative
    s. acute appendicitis
    s. acute inflammation
    s. appendicitis
    s. chronic inflammation
    s. chronic otitis media
    s. granulomatous inflammation
    s. inflammation

SVAS (supravalvular aortic stenosis)
sweat gland
    s. g. adenocarcinoma
    s. g. adenoma
    s. g. carcinoma
    s. g. tumor
Swediaur's disease
Sweet's syndrome
swelling
    albuminous s.
    arytenoid s.
    blenorrhagic s.
    Calabar's s.
    capsular s.
    cloudy s.
    fugitive s.
    genital s.
    glassy s.
    hunger s.
    Kamerun s's
    labial s.
    labioscrotal s.
    scrotal s.
    Soemmerring's crystalline s.
    tropical s's
    tympanic s.
    shite s.
Swift's disease
Swiss cheese hyperplasia
Swiss-type agammaglobulinemia
Swiss-type hypogammaglobulinemia
Swyer-James syndrome
sycosis
    s. barbae

Additional Entries

sycosis *(continued)*
    lupoid s.
    s. nuchae
    s. tarsi
    s. vulgaris
Sydenham's chorea
Sylvest's disease
symblepharon
    anterior s.
    posterior s.
    total s.
symblepharopterygium
symbrachydactyly
Symmers' disease
sympathetic ophthalmitis
sympathicoblastoma
sympodia
synarthrophysis
synathrosis
syncope
    cardiac s.
    carotid sinus s.
    exertional s.
    micturition s.
    postural s.
    swallow s.
    tussive s.
    vasovagal s.
syncytial endometritis
syndactyly
    complete s.
    complicated s.
    double s.
    partial s.
    simple s.
    single s.
    triple s.
syndesmitis

syndesmitis *(continued)*
    s. metatarsea
syndrome
    Aarskog s.
    Aase s.
    Abercrombie's s.
    abstinence s.
    Achard s.
    Achard-Thiers s.
    acquired immune defficiency s. (AIDS)
    acute brain s.
    acute radiation s.
    Adair-Dighton s.
    Adams-Stokes s.
    addisonian s.
    Adie's s.
    adiposogenital s.
    adrenogenital s.
    adult respiratory distress s. (ARDS)
    afferent loop s.
    aglossia-adactylia s.
    Ahumada-del Castillo s.
    Aicardi's s.
    Alajouanine's s.
    Albright's s.
    Aldrich's s.
    Alezzandrini's s.
    'Alice in Wonderland' s.
    Allemann's s.
    Alport's s.
    Alstrom s.
    amnesic s.
    amnestic s.
    amnestic-confabulatory s.
    amniotic infection s. of Blane

Additional Entries

syndrome *(continued)*
    amyostatic s.
    Andersen's s.
    Angelucci s.
    anorexia-cachexia s.
    anterior abdominal wall s.
    anterior chamber cleavage s.
    anterior cord s.
    anterior cornual s.
    anterior tibial compartment s.
    anticholinergic s.
    Anton's s.
    anxiety s.
    Apert s.
    argentaffinoma s.
    Arnold's nerve reflex cough s.
    Arnold-Chiari s.
    Ascher s.
    Asherman's s.
    Asherson's s.
    asplenia s.
    ataxia-telangiectasia s.
    auriculotemporal s.
    autoerythrocyte sensitization s.
    autoimmune polyendocrine-candidiasis s.
    Avellis' s.
    Axenfeld's s.
    Ayerza's s.
    Baastrup's s.
    Babinski's s.
    Babinski-Frohlich s.
    s. of Babinski-Nageotte

syndrome *(continued)*
    Babinski-Vaquez's s.
    BADS s.
    Bafverstedt's s.
    Balint's s.
    Baller-Gerold s.
    Bannwarth's s.
    Banti's s.
    Bardet-Biedl s.
    Barlow s.
    Barraquer-Simons' s.
    Barre-Guillain s.
    Barrett's s.
    Bart's s.
    Bartter's s.
    basal cell nevus s.
    Bassen-Kornzweig s.
    battered-child s.
    Bazex's s.
    Beals' s.
    Bearn-Kunkel s.
    Beau's s.
    Beckwith's s.
    Beckwith-Wiedemann s.
    Behcet's s.
    s. of Benedikt
    Bernard's s.
    Bernard-Sergent s.
    Bernard-Soulier s.
    Bernhardt-Roth s.
    Bernheim's s.
    Bertolotti's s.
    Bianchi's s.
    Biemond s., II
    Bjornstad's s.
    Blatin's s.
    blind loop s.
    Bloch-Sulzberger s.

Additional Entries

syndrome *(continued)*
    Bloom s.
    blue diaper s.
    Blum's s.
    body of Luys s.
    Boerhaave's s.
    Bonnier's s.
    Borjeson's s.
    Borjeson-Forssman-
       Lehmann s.
    Bouillaud's s.
    Bouveret's s.
    brachial s.
    Brachmann-de Lange s.
    bradycardia-tachycardia s.
    Brennemann's s.
    Briquet's s.
    Brissaud-Marie s.
    Brissaud-Sicard s.
    Bristowe's s.
    brittle bone s.
    brittle cornea s.
    Brock s.
    Brown's vertical retraction
       s.
    Brown-Sequard s.
    Bruns' s.
    Brunsting's s.
    Brushfield-Wyatt s.
    Buckely's s.
    Budd-Chiari s.
    Burger-Grutz s.
    Burnett's s.
    burning feet s.
    Buschke-Ollendorff s.
    Bywaters's s.
    Caffey's s.
    callosal s.

syndrome *(continued)*
    camptomelic s.
    Canada-Cronkhite s.
    Capgras' s.
    Caplan's s.
    Carpenter's s.
    s. of Cestan-Chenais
    Cestan-Raymond s.
    Cestan's s.
    Charcot's s.
    Charcot-Weiss-Barker s.
    Charlin's s.
    Chauffard's s.
    Chediak-Higashi s.
    Shauffard-Still s.
    Chediak-Steinbrinck-
       Higashi s.
    Cheney s.
    Chiari-Arnold s.
    Chiari-Budd s.
    Chiari-Frommel s.
    Chiari II s.
    Chiari's s.
    Chilaiditi's s.
    Chotzen's s.
    Christian's s.
    Christ-Siemens s.
    Christ-Siemens-Touraine
       s.
    Churg-Strauss s.
    Clarke-Hadfield s.
    Claude Bernard-Horner s.
    Claude's s.
    Clerambault-Kandinsky s.
    Clough and Richter's s.
    Clouston's s.
    Cockayne's s.
    Coffin-Lowry s.

Additional Entries

syndrome *(continued)*
    Coffin-Siris s.
    Cogan's s.
    Collet-Sicard s.
    Collet's s.
    Conn's s.
    Conradi's s.
    Cornelia de Lange's s.
    Costen's s.
    Cotard's s.
    Courvoisier-Terrier s.
    Crandall's s.
    Creutzfeldt-Jakob s.
    Crigler-Najjar s.
    Cronkhite-Canada s.
    Cronkhite's s.
    Cruveilhier-Baumgarten s.
    Cushing's s.
    Cyriax's s.
    DaCosta's s.
    Danbolt-Closs s.
    Dandy-Walker s.
    Danlos s.
    Debre-Semelaigne s.
    de Clerambault s.
    Degos' s.
    Dejerine-Klumpke s.
    s. of Dejerine-Roussy
    Dejerine's s.
    Dejerine-Sottas s,
    de Lange's s.
    del Castillo s.
    Dennie-Marfan s.
    De Sanctis-Cacchione s.
    de Toni-Fanconi s.
    DiGeorge's s.
    Dighton-Adair s.
    Di Guglielmo s.

syndrome *(continued)*
    Donohue's s.
    Down's s.
    Dresbach's s.
    Dressler's s.
    Duane's s.
    Dubin-Johnson s.
    Dubin-Sprinz s.
    Dubois' s.
    Dubreuil-Chambardel s.
    Duchenne-Erb s.
    Duchenne's s.
    Duplay's s.
    Dupre's s.
    Dyggve-Melchior-Clausen s.
    Dyke-Davidoff s.
    Eagle s.
    Eales's s.
    Eaton-Lambert s.
    Eddowes' s.
    Edwards-Patau s.
    Edwards' s.
    Ehlers-Danlos s.
    Eisenlohr's s.
    Eisenmenger's s.
    Ekbom s.
    Ellis-van Creveld s.
    Epstein's s.
    Erb's s.
    Faber's s.
    Fallot's s.
    Fanconi's s.
    Farber's s.
    Farber-Uzman s.
    Favre-Racouchot s.
    Felty's s.
    Fiessinger-Leroy-Reiter s.

Additional Entries

syndrome *(continued)*
    Fiessinger's s.
    Figueira's s.
    Fisher's s.
    Fitz-Hugh-Curtis s.
    Fitz's s.
    Flynn-Aird s.
    Foix's s.
    Forbes-Albright s.
    Forney's s.
    Forssman's carotid s.
    Foster Kennedy s.
    Foville's s.
    Fraley s.
    Franceschetti-Jadassohn s.
    Franceschetti s.
    Francois' s.
    Fraser's s.
    Freeman-Sheldon s.
    Frenkel's anterior ocular traumatic s.
    Frey's s.
    Friderichsen-Waterhouse s.
    Friedmann's vasomotor s.
    Frolich's s.
    Frommel-Chiari s.
    Fuchs's s.
    Gailliard's s.
    Ganser's s.
    Gardner-Diamond s.
    Gardner's s.
    Gasser's s.
    Gerstmann's s.
    Gianotti-Crosti s.
    Gilbert's s.
    Gilles de la Tourette's s.
    Glanzmann-Riniker s.

syndrome *(continued)*
    Goldberg-Maxwell s.
    Goltz-Gorlin s.
    Goltz's s.
    Goodpasture's s.
    Good's s.
    Gopalan's s.
    Gorlin-Goltz s.
    Gorlin-Psaume s.
    Gorlin's s.
    Gougerot-Carteaud s.
    Gougerot-Nulock-Houwer s.
    Gowers' s.
    Gradenigo's s.
    Graham Little s.
    Greig's s.
    Gronblad-Strandberg s.
    Gruber's s.
    Gubler's s.
    Guillain-Barre s.
    Gunn's s.
    Haber's s.
    Hadfield-Clarke s.
    Hakim's s.
    Hallermann-Streiff s.
    Hallermann-Streiff-Francois s.
    Hallervorden s.
    Hallervorden-Spatz s.
    Hallgren's s.
    Hallopeau-Siemens s.
    Hamman-Rich s.
    Hanhart's s.
    Hanot-Chauffard s.
    Harada's s.
    Hare's s.
    Harris' s.

Additional Entries

syndrome *(continued)*
    Hartnup s.
    Hassin's s.
    Hayem-Widal s.
    Heerfordt's s.
    Hegglin's s.
    Heidenhaim's s.
    Helwig-Larssen s.
    Hench-Rosenberg s.
    Henoch-Schonlein s.
    Herrmann's s.
    Hines-Bannick s.
    Hoffmann-Werdnig s.
    Holmes-Adie s.
    Holt-Oram s.
    Homen's s.
    Horner-Bernard s.
    Horner's s.
    Horton's s.
    Houssay s.
    Hunter-Hurler s.
    Hunter's s.
    Hunt's s.
    Hurler-Pfaundler s.
    Hurler's s.
    Hutchinson s.
    Irvine's s.
    Ivemark's s.
    Jaccoud's s.
    Jackson's s.
    Jacod's s.
    Jadassohn-Lewandowsky s.
    Jaffe-Lichtenstein s.
    Jahnke's s.
    Jervell and Lange-Nielsen s.
    Jeune's s.

syndrome *(continued)*
    Job's s.
    Kallmann's s.
    Kanner's s.
    Kasabach-Merritt s.
    Kast's s.
    Kearns' s.
    Kennedy's s.
    Kiloh-Nevin s.
    Kimmelstiel-Wilson s.
    Kinsbourne s.
    Klauder's s.
    Kleine-Levin s.
    Klinefelter's s.
    Klippel-Feil s.
    Klippel-Trenaunay-Weber s.
    Klumpke-Dejerine s.
    Kluver-Bucy s.
    Kneist s.
    Kocher-Debre-Semelaigne s.
    Kocher's s.
    Koenig's s.
    Koerber-Salus-Elschnig s.
    Konig's s.
    Korsakoff's s.
    Krabbe's s.
    Krause's s.
    Kunkel's s.
    Kuskokwim s.
    Laband's s.
    Labbe's neurocirculatory s.
    Ladd's s.
    Lambert-Eaton s.
    Landry's s.
    Laubry-Soulle s.

Additional Entries

syndrome *(continued)*
 Launois' s.
 Launois-Cleret s.
 Laurence-Biedl s.
 Laurence-Moon s.
 Laurence-Moon-Bardet-
  Biedl s.
 Laurence-Moon-Biedl s.
 Lawen-Roth s.
 Lawford's s.
 Lawrence-Seip s.
 Lennox's s.
 Lenz's s.
 Leredde's s.
 Leriche's s.
 Leri-Weill s.
 Lermoyez's s.
 Lesch-Nyhan s.
 Levi's s.
 Levy-Roussy s.
 Leyden-Moebius s.
 Lhermitte and McAlpine s.
 Libman-Sacks s.
 Lichtheim's s.
 Lightwood's s.
 Lignac-Fanconi s.
 Liganc's s.
 Loffler's s.
 Looser-Milkman s.
 Lorain-Levi s.
 Louis-Bar s.
 Lowe's s.
 Lowe-Terrey-MacLachlan s.
 Lown-Ganong-Levine s.
 Lucey-Driscoll s.
 Lyell's s.
 Mackenzie's s.

syndrome *(continued)*
 Macleod's s.
 Maffucci's s.
 Malin's s.
 Mallory-Weiss s.
 Maranon's s.
 Marchesani's s.
 Marcus Gunn's s.
 Marfan's s.
 Margolis s.
 Marinesco-Garland s.
 Marie-Bamberger s.
 Marie-Robinson s.
 Marinesco-Sjogren's s.
 Maroteaux-Lamy s.
 Marshall's s.
 Martorell's s.
 Mauriac s.
 Mayer-Rokitansky-Kuster s.
 McCune-Albright s.
 Meckel-Gruber s.
 Meckel's s.
 Melkersson-Rosenthal s.
 Melkersson's s.
 Melnick-Needles s.
 Mendelson's s.
 Mengert's shock s.
 Meniere's s.
 Menkes' s.
 Meyenburg-Altherr-Uehlinger s.
 Meyer-Schwickerath and Weyers s.
 Milkman's s.
 Millard-Gubler s.
 Minkowski-Chauffard s.
 Minot-von Willebrand s.

Additional Entries

syndrome *(continued)*
- Mobius' s.
- Monakow's s.
- Morel's s.
- Morgagni-Adams-Stokes s.
- Morgagni's s.
- Morgagni-Stewart-Morel s.
- Morquio's s.
- Morquio-Ullrich s.
- Morris s.
- Morton's s.
- Morvan's s.
- Mosse's s.
- Mounier-Kuhn s.
- Mucha-Habermann s.
- Muckle-Wells s.
- Munchausen's s.
- Murchison-Sanderson s.
- Naegeli's s.
- Naffziger's s.
- Nelson's s.
- Netherton's s.
- Nezelof's s.
- Nieden's s.
- Noack's s.
- Nonne-Milroy-Meige s.
- Nonne's s.
- Noonan's s.
- Nothnagel's s.
- Ogilvie's s.
- Ostrum-Furst s.
- Pancoast's s.
- Papillon-Leage and Psaume s.
- Papillon-Lefevre s.

syndrome *(continued)*
- Parinaud's oculoglandular s.
- Parinaud's s.
- parkinsonian s.
- Parry-Romberg s.
- Paterson-Brown-Kelly s.
- Paterson-Kelly s.
- Paterson's s.
- Pellizzi's s.
- Pendred's s.
- Pepper s.
- Peutz-Jeghers s.
- Peutz s.
- Pfeiffer's s.
- Picchini's s.
- pickwickian s.
- Pierre Robin s.
- Plummer-Vinson s.
- Poland's s.
- Polhemus-Schafer-Ivemark s.
- Potter's s.
- Prader-Willi s.
- pseudo-Turner's s.
- Putnam-Dana s.
- Ramsay Hunt s.
- Raymond-Cestan s.
- Refetoff s.
- Reifenstein's s.
- Reiter's s.
- Renpenning's s.
- Reye's s.
- Richards-Rundle s.
- Richter's s.
- Rieger's s.
- Riley-Day s.
- Riley-Smith s.

Additional Entries

syndrome *(continued)*
   Roaf's s.
   Robert's s.
   Robinow's s.
   Robin's s.
   Rokitansky-Kuster-Hauser s.
   Romano-Ward s.
   Romberg's s.
   Rosenbach's s.
   Rosenthal-Kloepfer s.
   Rosenthal's s.
   Rosewater's s.
   Rothmann-Makai s.
   Rothmund-Thomson s.
   Roth's s.
   Rotor's s.
   Rotter's s.
   Roussy-Dejerine s.
   Roussy-Levy s.
   Rovsing s.
   Rubinstein's s.
   Rubinstein-Taybi s.
   Rud's s.
   Russell's s.
   Rust's s.
   Sabin-Feldman s.
   Saethre-Chotzen s.
   Sanchez Salorio s.
   Sanfilippo's s.
   Schafer's s.
   Schanz's s.
   Schaumann's s.
   Scheie's s.
   Schirmer's s.
   Schmid-Fraccaro s.
   Schmidt's s.
   Schuller's s.

syndrome *(continued)*
   Schultz s.
   Schwartz s.
   Seckel's s.
   Selye s.
   Senear-Usher s.
   Sertoli-cell-only s.
   Sezary reticulosis s.
   Sezary s.
   Sheehan's s.
   Shwachman s.
   Shwachman-Diamond s.
   Shy-Drager s.
   Sicard's s.
   Silverskiold's s.
   Silver's s.
   Silvestrini-Corda s.
   Sjogren-Larsson s.
   Sluder's s.
   Smith-Lemli-Opitz s.
   Sohval-Soffer s.
   Sorsby's s.
   Sotos' s.
   Sotos' s. of cerebral gigantism
   Spens's s.
   Speransky-Richen-Siegmund s.
   Sprinz-Dubin s.
   Sprinz-Nelson s.
   Spurway s.
   Steele-Richardson-Olszewski s.
   Steinbrocker's s.
   Steiner's s.
   Stein-Leventhal s.
   Stevens-Johnson s.
   Stewart-Morel s.

Additional Entries

syndrome *(continued)*
    Stewart-Treves s.
    Stickler s.
    Still-Chauffard s.
    Stilling s.
    Stilling-Turk-Duane s.
    Stokvis-Talma s.
    Stryker-Halbeisen s.
    Sturge-Kalischer-Weber s.
    Sturge's s.
    Sturge-Weber s.
    Sudeck-Leriche s.
    Sulzberger-Garbe s.
    Sweet's s.
    Takayasu's s.
    Taussig-Bing s.
    Terry's s.
    Thibierge-Weissenbach s.
    Thiele s.
    Thorn's s.
    Thornwaldt's s.
    Tietze's s.
    Timme's s.
    Tolosa-Hunt s.
    Torre's s.
    Torsten-Sjogren's s.
    Touraine-Solente-Gole s.
    Treacher Collins s.
    Troisier's s.
    Trousseau's s.
    Turcot s.
    Turner's s.
    Uehlinger's s.
    Ullrich-Turner s.
    Ulysses s.
    Usher's s.
    van Buchem's s.
    van der Hoeve's s.

syndrome *(continued)*
    Van der Woude's s.
    Verner-Morrison s.
    Vernet's s.
    Villaret's s.
    Vinson-Plummer s.
    Vinson's s.
    Vogt-Koyanagi s.
    Vogt's s.
    Vohwinkel's s.
    von Willebrand's s.
    Waardenburg's s.
    Wallenberg's s.
    Waterhouse-Friderichsen s.
    s. of Weber
    Weber-Cockayne s.
    Weber-Dubler s.
    Wegener's s.
    Weill-Marchesani s.
    Weil's s.
    Werdnig-Hoffmann s.
    Wermer's s.
    Werner's s.
    Wernicke-Korsakoff s.
    Wernicke's s.
    West's s.
    Weyers' oligodactyly s.
    Weyers-Thier s.
    Widal s.
    Wildervanck s.
    Willebrand's s.
    Williams-Campbell s.
    Williams s.
    Wilson-Mikity s.
    Wilson's s.
    Winter's s.
    Wiskott-Aldrich s.

Additional Entries

syndrome *(continued)*
    Wolff-Parkinson-White s.
    Wolf-Hirschhorn s.
    Wolfram s.
    Wright's s.
    Young's s.
    Zellweger s.
    Zieve s.
    Zollinger-Ellison s.
synechia
    annular s.
    anterior s.
    circular s.
    s. pericardii
    posterior s.
    total anterior s.
    total posterior s.
    s. vulvae
Syngamus
    S. laryngeus
    S. trachea
synophthalmia
Synosternus
    S. pallidus
synostosis
    radioulnar s.
    sagittal s.
    tarsal s.
    tribasilar s.
synovioma
synovitis
    acute serous s.
    bursal s.
    dendritic s.
    dry s.
    fungus s.
    localized nodular s.
    pigmented villonodular s.

synovitis *(continued)*
    proliferative s.
    purulent s.
    serous s.
    s. sicca
    simple s.
    tendinous s.
    vaginal s.
    vibration s.
    villonodular s.
syphilis
    cardiovascular s.
    cerebrospinal s.
    congenital s.
    early s.
    early latent s.
    endemic s.
    gummatous s.
    late s.
    late benign s.
    latent s.
    meningovascular s.
    nonvenereal s.
    parenchymatous s.
    primary s.
    secondary s.
    tertiary s.
syphilitic
    s. aneurysm
    s. aortitis
syringadenoma
    papillary s.
syringocystadenoma
    s. papilliferum
syringoencephalomyelia
syringoma
    chondroid s.
syringomyelia

Additional Entries

syringomyelocele
systemic
    s. familial primary
        amyloidosis
    s. lupus erythematosus
    s. primary amyloidosis

systemic *(continued)*
    s. reticuloendotheliosis
    s. sclerosis
systolic
    s. hypertension
    s. murmur

Additional Entries

T

T. (Taenia; Treponema; Trichophyton; Trypanosoma)
taboparesis
tachycardia
    atrial t.
    junctional t.
    nodal t.
    paroxysmal auricular t.
    paroxysmal ventricular t.
    ventricular t.
tachypnea
tactile hypesthesia
TAD (thoracic asphyxiant dystrophy)
Taenia
    T. africana
    T. bremneri
    T. canina
    T. confusa
    T. diminuta
    T. echinococcus
    T. lata
    T. murina
    T. nana
    T. philippina
    T. saginata
    T. solium
    T. taeniaeformis
Taeniarhynchus
taeniasis
Takayasu's syndrome
Tangier disease
tapeworm
    beef t.
    dwarf t.

tapeworm *(continued)*
    fish t.
    pork t.
TAPVD (total anomalous pulmonary venous drainage)
Taussig-Bing syndrome
Tay-Sachs disease
TB (tuberculosis)
TBM (tuberculosis meningitis)
TCI (transient cerebral ischemia)
TCIE (transient cerebral ischemic episode)
Te (tetanus)
telangiectasia
    hereditary hemorrhagic t.
telangiectasis
tendinitis
tenostosis
tenosynovitis
    t. acuta purulenta
    adhesive t.
    t. crepitans
    gonorrheal t.
    t. granulosa
    t. hypertrophica
    infectious t.
    nodular t.
    t. serosa chronica
    t. stenosans
    tuberculous t.
    villonodular t.
    villous t.
tenovaginitis
teratocarcinoma
teratoma

Additional Entries

teratoma *(continued)*
    adult cystic t.
    benign t.
    embryonal t.
    malignant t.
    monodermal t.
    solid t.
tertiary
    t. syphilis
Teschen virus
testicular
    t. agenesis
    t. dysgenesis
    t. feminization
    t. tumor
tetanus
    t. bacillus
tetany
tetraplegia
Tetratrichomonas
    T. buccalis
    T. hominis
Tfm (testicular feminization syndrome)
thalassemia
    hemoglobin t.
    heterozygous t.
    homozygous t.
    t. intermedia
    t. major
    t. minor
    mixed t.
    sickle-cell t.
    t. trait
thallitoxicosis
thecitis
thecoma
thecomatosis

Theiler's virus
Thelazia
    T. callipaeda
thermal
    t. death point
    t. death time
    t. hypesthesia
Thermoactinomyces
    T. vulgaris
third degree
    t. d. burn
    t. d. frostbite
    t. d. heart block
    t. d. radiation injury
thoracoceloschisis
thoracocyllosis
thoracocyrtosis
thoracodynia
thoracogastroschisis
thoracomyodynia
thoracoschisis
thoracostenosis
thrill
    aneurysmal t.
    aortic t.
    diastolic t.
    hydatid t.
    presystolic t.
    systolic t.
thrombasthenia
    Glanzmann-Naegeli t.
    Glanzmann's t.
thromboangiitis obliterans
thromboarteritis
    t. purulenta
thrombocythemia
    hemorrhagic t.
    primary t.

Additional Entries

thrombocytic
    t. leukemia
thrombocytopathy
thrombocytopenia
thrombocytopenic purpura
    autoimmune t. p.
    idopathic t. p.
    thrombotic t. p.
thrombocytosis
thromboembolism
thromboendarteritis
thromboendocarditis
thrombonecrosis
    arteriolar t.
thrombopathy
    constitutional t.
thrombophlebitis
    migrating t.
thrombosed
    t. aneurysm
    t. arteriosclerotic aneurysm
    t. hemorrhoids
thrombosis
    agonal t.
    cardiac t.
    cerebral t.
    coronary t.
    dilatation t.
    marantic t.
    mesenteric t.
    placental t.
    propagating t.
    puerperal t.
    traumatic t.
    venous t.
thrombotic

thrombotic *(continued)*
    t. nonbacterial endocarditis
    t. occlusion
    t. thrombocytopenic purpura
thrombus
    canalized t.
    marantic t.
    mural t.
    old t.
    organized t.
    platelet t.
    recent t.
    tumor t.
thrush
thymic
    t. carcinoma
    t. leukemia
thymoma
    epithelial t.
    lymphocytic t.
thymopathy
thyroglossal
    t. duct cyst
thyroid
    t. crisis
    t. endocrine disorder
    t. tumor
thyroiditis
    de Quervain's t.
    granulomatous t.
    Hashimoto's t.
    induced t.
    ligneous t.
    Riedel's t.
    subacute t.
thyrosis

Additional Entries

thyrotoxicosis
    t. factitia
TIA (transient ischemic attack)
tick
    t.-borne fever, African
    t. fever, Colorado
    t. paralysis
Tietze's syndrome
tinnitus
TIS (tumor in situ)
Tityus serrulatus
TNF (tumor necrosis factor)
TOA (tubo-ovarian abscess)
tonic clonic attack
tonsillitis
    caseous t.
    catarrhal t., acute
    catarrhal t., chronic
    diphtherial t.
    erythematous t.
    follicular t.
    herpetic t.
    lacunar t.
    t. lenta
    lingual t.
    mycotic t.
    parenchymatous t.
    preglottic t.
    pustular t.
    streptococcal t.
    superficial t.
    suppurative t.
    Vincent's t.
TORCH (toxoplasmosis, rubella, cytomegalovirus and herpes simplex)
Tornwaldt's disease
torticollis

torticollis *(continued)*
    congenital t.
    dermatogenic t.
    fixed t.
    hysteric t.
    intermittent t.
    labyrinthine t.
    mental t.
    myogenic t.
    neurogenic t.
    ocular t.
    reflex t.
    rheumatoid t.
    spasmodic t.
    spurious t.
    symptomatic t.
Torulopsis
    T. glabrata
torulopsosis
torulosis
Touraine-Solente-Gole syndrome
Tourette's disease
toxanemia
toxemia
    alimentary t.
    ecclamptic t.
    hydatid t.
    preeclamptic t.
    t. of pregnancy
toxic
    t. adenoma
    t. cirrhosis
    t. dermatitis
    t. erythema
    t. goiter
    t. granulation
    t. nephrosis

Additional Entries

toxic *(continued)*
    t. shock syndrome
toxicopathy
toxicosis
    endogenic t.
    exogenic t.
    gestational t.
    hemorrhagic capillary t.
    proteinogenous t.
    retention t.
toxinemia
toxinosis
Toxocara
    T. canis
    T. cati
    T. mystax
toxocariasis
    human t.
Toxoplasma
    T. gondii
    T. pyrogenes
toxoplasmosis
TPA (Treponema pallidum)
TPH (transplacental hemorrhage)
trabecular
    t. adenocarcinoma
    t. adenoma
    t. carcinoma
trachealgia
tracheitis
trachelagra
trachelematoma
trachelism
trachelocele
trachelocyllosis
trachelocystitis
trachelodynia

trachelokyphosis
trachelomyitis
tracheloschisis
tracheoaerocele
tracheobronchitis
tracheomalacia
tracheopathia
    t. osteoplastica
tracheopyosis
tracheorrhagia
tracheoschisis
tracheostenosis
trachoma
    Arlt's t.
    Turck's t.
    t. virus
    t. of vocal bands
Trachybdella bistriata
traction
    t. atrophy
    t. diverticulum
trait
    sickle cell t.
tramitis
transient
    t. hypogammaglobulinemia
    t. ischemic attack
transitional cell
    t. c. carcinoma
    t. c. papilloma
transudate
    acute inflammatory t.
transverse
    t. myelitis
    t. myelopathy
Treacher Collins syndrome
tremor

Additional Entries

tremor *(continued)*
    action t.
    arsenic t.
    coarse t.
    continuous t.
    t. cordis
    darkness t.
    epidemic t.
    epileptoid t.
    essential t.
    familial t.
    fibrillary t.
    fine t.
    forced t.
    hereditary essential t.
    Hunt's t.
    intention t.
    intermittent t.
    kinetic t.
    t. linguae
    t. mercurialis
    metallic t.
    passive t.
    persistent t.
    t. potatorum
    rest t.
    senile t.
    striocerebellar t.
    toxic t.
    volitional t.
trench
    t. fever
    t. foot
    t. mouth
Treponema
    T. buccale
    T. calligyrum
    T. carateum

Treponema *(continued)*
    T. macrodentium
    T. microdentium
    T. mucosum
    T. orale
    T. pallidum
    T. pertenue
    T. pintae
    T. refringens
    T. scoliodontum
    T. vincentii
treponematosis
TRIC (trachoma-inclusion conjunctivitis)
Trichinella
    T. spiralis
trichinosis
Trichobilharzia
trichocephaliasis
trichoepithelioma
Trichomonas
    T. buccalis
    T. hominis
    T. intestinalis
    T. pulmonalis
    T. vaginalis
trichomoniasis
trichomycosis
    t. axillaris
    t. chromatica
    t. favosa
    t. rubra
trichonodosis
Trichophyton
    T. concentricum
    T. crateriforme
    T. epilans
    T. ferrugineum

Additional Entries

Trichophyton *(continued)*
    T. gallinae
    T. glabrum
    T. gourvilii
    T. gypseum
    T. megninii
    T. mentagrophytes
    T. purpureum
    T. rosaceum
    T. rubrum
    T. sabouraudi
    T. schoenleini
    T. simii
    T. sulfureum
    T. tonsurans
    T. verrucosum
    T. violaceum
trichophytosis
trichorrhexis
    t. nodosa
Trichosporon
    T. beigelii
    T. cutaneum
    T. giganteum
    T. pedrosianum
trichosporosis
trichostrongyliasis
Trichostrongylus
    T. axei
    T. brevis
    T. colubriformis
    T. instabilis
    T. orientalis
    T. probolurus
    T. vitrinus
trichuriasis
Trichuris
    T. trichiura

trigonitis
trismus
Trombicula
    T. akamushi
    T. alfreddugesi
    T. autumnalis
    T. deliensis
    T. irritans
    T. pallida
    T. scutellaris
    T. tsalsahuatl
    T. vandersandi
trombiculiasis
Tromner's sign
trophoblastic
    gestational t. disease
    t. neoplasia
trophoneurosis
    facial t.
    lingual t.
    muscular t.
    t. of Romberg
trophonosis
trophopathy
Trousseau's sign
Trypanosoma
    T. ariari
    T. brucei
    T. castellani
    T. cruzi
    T. gambiense
    T. hominis
    T. nigeriense
    T. rangeli
    T. rhodesiense
    T. triatomae
    T. ugandense
trypanosomiasis

Additional Entries

trypanosomiasis *(continued)*
    Gambian t.
    Rhodesian t.
TSD (Tay-Sachs disease)
tsutsugamushi disease
tuberculitis
tuberculocele
tuberculoderma
tuberculoid granuloma
tuberculoma
    t. en plaque
tuberculosilicosis
tuberculosis
    central nervous system t.
    t. cutis verrucosa
    endobronchial t.
    extrapulmonary t.
    gastrointestinal t.
    healed t.
    inactive t.
    laryngeal t.
    miliary t.
    pericardial t.
    pleural t.
    primary t.
    pulmonary t.
    secondary t.
    tracheobronchial t.
tuberculous meningitis
tuberous sclerosis
tubular
    t. interstitial nephritis
    Pick's t. adenoma
tubulointerstitial nephropathy
tubulonecrosis
tubulorrhexis
tularemia
    oculoglandular t.

tularemia *(continued)*
    pneumonic t.
    typhoidal t.
    ulceroglandular t.
tumor
    Abrikosov's t.
    acoustic nerve t.
    acute splenic t.
    adenoid t.
    adenomatoid t.
    adipose t.
    amyloid t.
    t. angiogenesis
    benign t.
    Brenner's t.
    Brooke's t.
    brown t.
    Brown-Pearce t.
    Burkitt's t.
    Buschke-Lowenstein t.
    carcinoid t. of bronchus
    carotid body t.
    cartilaginous t.
    Codman's t.
    t. colli
    colloid t.
    connective tissue t.
    craniopharyngeal duct t.
    cystic t.
    dermoid t.
    desmoid t.
    eiloid t.
    t. embolus
    embryonal t.
    endobronchial t.
    epithelial t., benign
    Ewing's t.
    fatty t.

Additional Entries

tumor *(continued)*
    fibrocellular t.
    fibroid t.
    fungating t.
    giant cell t.
    giant cell t. of tendon sheath
    glomus t.
    granular cell t.
    granulosa cell t.
    granulosa-theca cell t.
    Grawitz's t.
    hilar cell t.
    histoid t.
    Hortega cell t.
    hourglass t.
    Hurthle cell t.
    infiltrating t.
    islet cell t.
    Jensen's t.
    Krukenberg's t.
    Leydig-Sertoli cell t.
    lipoid cell t. of ovary
    malignant t.
    mast cell t.
    melanotic neuroectodermal cell t.
    metastatic t.
    migrated t.
    mixed t.
    monoclonal t.
    mucous t.
    necrosis t.
    neuroepithelial t.
    ovarian t.
    Pancoast's t.
    papillary t.
    Perlmann's t.

tumor *(continued)*
    plasma cell t.
    polyclonal t.
    Pott's puffy t.
    pregnancy t.
    premalignant fibroepithelial t.
    pulmonary sulcus t.
    Rathke's pouch t.
    recurring digital fibrous t's of childhood
    Sertoli-Leydig cell t.
    Schwann cell t.
    Sertoli cell t.
    sheath t.
    theca cell t.
    thrombus t.
    true t.
    turban t.
    varicose t.
    vascular t.
    villous t.
    Warthin's t.
    white t.
    Wilms' t.
Tunga
    T. penetrans
tungiasis
turban tumor
Turcot's syndrome
Turner's syndrome
tympanomastoiditis
tympanosclerosis
typhoid
    t. bacillus
    t. fever
typhus
    amarillic t.

Additional Entries

typhus *(continued)*
    endemic t.
    epidemic t.
    louse-borne t.
    murine t.

typhus *(continued)*
    recrudescent t.
    scrub t.
tyrosinemia
tyrosinosis
tyrosinuria

Additional Entries

U

UC (ulcerative colitis)
U-cell lymphoma
Uganda S virus
Uhl's anomaly
UIP (usual interstitial pneumonitis)
UL (undifferentiated lymphoma)
ulatrophy
    atrophic u.
    calcic u.
    ischemic u.
ulcer
    acute u.
    acute hemorrhagic u.
    amebic u.
    aphthous u.
    Barrett's u.
    catarrhal corneal u.
    chancroidal u.
    chronic u.
    corneal u.
    Curling's u.
    Cushing's u.
    decubitus u.
    diabetic u.
    duodenal u.
    focal u.
    gastric u.
    healed u.
    hemorrhagic u.
    Hunner's u.
    marginal u.
    penetrating u.
    peptic u.
    perforated u.

ulcer *(continued)*
    serpiginous u.
    stasis u.
    stercoraceous u.
    stomal u.
    trophic u.
    varicose u.
    venereal u.
ulcerative
    u. colitis
    u. cystitis
    u. inflammation
ulcerogangrenous
ulcerogenic tumor
ulemorrhagia
ulerythema
    u. ophryogenes
Ullrich-Feichtiger syndrome
Ullrich's syndrome
Ullrich-Turner syndrome
ulocace
ulocarcinoma
uloglossitis
ulorrhagia
ulorrhea
uncinariasis
uncinate
    u. epilepsy
unconsciousness
Underwood's disease
undifferentiated
    u. adenocarcinoma
    u. carcinoma
    u. epidermoid carcinoma
    u. lymphoma

Additional Entries

_____
_____
_____
_____

undifferentiated *(continued)*
    u. sarcoma
    u. squamous cell
      carcinoma
Undritz anomaly
undulant fever
unilocular
    u. cyst
    u. echinococcosis
    u. hydatid
unresolved
    u. hepatitis
    u. lobar pneumonia
    u. pneumonia
Unschuld's sign
uranoschisis
uranostaphyloschisis
urarthritis
Urbach-Oppenheim disease
Urbach-Wiethe disease
URD (upper respiratory disease)
uremia
uremic
    u. colitis
    u. inflammation
    u. pericarditis
    u. pneumonia
ureteralgia
ureterectasis
ureteritis
    u. cystica
    u. glanularis
ureterocele
    ectopic u.
ureterolithiasis
ureteropathy
ureteropyelitis
ureteropyelonephritis
ureteropyosis
ureterorrhagia
ureterostenosis
urethral
    u. obstruction
    u. tumor
urethritis
    u. cystica
    follicular u.
    u. glandularis
    gonorrheal u.
    gouty u.
    granular u.
urethroblenorrhea
urethrocele
urethrocystitis
urethrodynia
urethrophraxis
urethrorrhagia
urethrorrhea
urethrostaxis
urethrostenosis
urethrotrigonitis
urhidrosis
URI (upper respiratory infection)
uricacidemia
uricosuria
urinary tract infection
urine
    chylous u.
    diabetic u.
    gouty u.
    milky u.
    residual u.
urocystitis
urodynia
uroedema

Additional Entries

urohematonephrosis
urolithiasis
uronephrosis
uropyonephrosis
urorrhagia
urorrhea
urochesis
urosepsis
URTI (upper respiratory tract infection)
urticaria
    aquagenic u.
    cholinergic u.
    factitious u.
    giant u.
    papular u.
    u. perstans
    u. pigmentosa
    solar u.
Uruma virus
usual interstitial pneumonia
uterus
    u. acollis

uturus *(continued)*
    u. arcuatus
    u. bicameratus vetularum
    ribbon u.
UTI (urinary tract infection)
utriculitis
uveitis
    anterior u.
    Forster's u.
    granulomatous u.
    lens-induced u.
    nongranulomatous u.
    phacoantigenic u.
    phacotoxic u.
    posterior u.
    sympathetic u.
    toxoplasmic u.
    tuberculous u.
uveomeningitis
uveoparotid fever
uveoscleritis
uvulitis
uvuloptosis

Additional Entries

Additional Entries

V

vagabond's
  disease
  melanosis
vaginitis
  emphysematous v.
vaginomycosis
valley fever
valvular
  v. atresia
  v. incompetence
  v. malformation
  v. stenosis
  v. tissue embolus
valvulitis
  rheumatic v.
van Bogaert's disease
van Buren's disease
Vaquex-Osler disease
Vaquez's disease
varicella
  v. virus
  v. zoster
  v.-zoster virus
varicelliform eruption
  Kaposi's v. e.
varices
  esophageal v.
varicocele
varicose
  v. ulcer
  v. vein
variola virus
vascular
  v. anomaly
  v. hemophilia

vascular *(continued)*
  v. leiomyoma
vasculitis
  necrotizing v.
  nodular v.
  segmented hyalinizing v.
vasitis
vasomotor
  v. dysfunction
  v. hypotonia
  v. rhinitis
VD (venereal disease)
VDG (venereal disease - gonorrhea)
vegetative endocarditis
venous thrombosis
ventricular
  v. fibrillation
  v. premature beat
  v. premature contraction
  v. premature depolarization
  v. septal defect
  v. tachycardia
Verner-Morrison syndrome
Vernet's syndrome
verruca
  v. peruana
  v. plana
  v. plantaris
  v. seborrheica
  v. virus
  v. vulgaris
verrucal
  v. atypical endocarditis

Additional Entries

verrucal *(continued)*
    v. nonbacterial
        endocarditis
verrucous
    v. carcinoma
    v. endocarditis
    v. papilloma
vertebral basilar artery syndrome
vertigo
vesicolithiasis
vesicular
    v. acute inflammation
    v. emphysema
    v. granulomatous
        inflammation
    v. inflammation
    v. pharyngitis
    v. stomatitis
vesiculitis
VF (ventricular fibrillation)
VG (ventricular gallop)
VH (viral hepatitis)
VHD (viral hematodepressive disease)
vibratory sense loss
Vibrio
    v. alginolyticus
    v. bubulus
    v. cholerae
    v. cholerae-asiaticae
    v. coli
    v. comma
    v. danubicus
    v. eltor
    v. fecalis
    v. fetus
    v. finkleri
    v. ghinda

Vibrio *(continued)*
    v. jejuni
    v. massauah
    v. metschnikovii
    v. niger
    v. parahaemolyticus
    v. phosphorescens
    v. proteus
    v. septicus
    v. sputorum
    v. tyrogenus
    v. vulnificis
vibriosis
vicarious menstruation
Vidal's disease
Villaret's syndrome
villonodular
    v. pigmented synovitis
    v. pigmented
        tenosynovitis
villous
    v. adenoma
    v. papilloma
    v. tenosynovitis
Vincent's
    angina
    stomatitis
Vinson-Plummer syndrome
viral
    v. hepatitis
    v. pneumonia
viremia
viridans streptococcus
virilizing syndrome
virus
    animal v's
    APC v.
    apeu v.

Additional Entries

virus *(continued)*
    arbor v's, groups A, B, C, unclassified
    Argentinian hemorrhagic fever v.
    attenuated v.
    Australian X disease v.
    Australian X encephalitis v.
    bacterial v.
    biundulant milk fever v.
    Brunhilde v.
    Bunyamwera v.
    Bwamba fever v.
    C v.
    CA v.
    Cache Valley v.
    California encephalitis v.
    Central European encephalitis v.
    chickenpox v.
    chikungunya fever v.
    Coe v.
    Colorado tick fever v.
    Columbia SK v.
    common cold v.
    coryza v.
    cowpox v.
    Coxsackie v., A, type 1; B, type I
    Crimean hemorrhagic fever v.
    croup-associated v.
    cytomegalic inclusion disease v.
    dengue v., types 1, 2, 3, 4
    dephasic meningoencephalitis v.

virus *(continued)*
    diphasic milk fever v.
    distemper v.
    eastern equine encephalomyelitis v.
    Ebola v.
    EBV v.
    ECBO v.
    ECDO v.
    ECHO v., type 1, type 12, type 28
    ECMO v.
    ECSO v.
    ecthyma infectiosum v.
    EEE v.
    EMC v.
    encephalomyocarditis v.
    enteric cytopathogenic human orphan v.
    entomopox v.
    epidemic keratoconjunctivitis v.
    epidemic parotitis v.
    Epstein-Barr v.
    erythema infectiosum v.
    exanthem subitum v.
    fifth disease v.
    filterable v.
    fixed v.
    foot-and-mouth disease v., types A, B, C
    German measles v.
    Guama v.
    Guaroa v.
    hemadsorption v., types 1, 2
    hepatitis v.
    herpangina v.

Additional Entries

virus *(continued)*
- herpes simplex v., I, II
- herpes zoster v.
- human T cell leukemia-lymphoma v.
- Ilheus v.
- inclusion conjunctivitis v.
- infectious hepatitis v.
- influenza v., types A, B, C
- Itaqui v.
- Japanese B encephalitis v.
- JH v.
- Junin v.
- Kumba v.
- Kyasanur Forest disease v.
- Lansing v.
- Lassa v.
- latent v.
- LCM v.
- Leon v.
- lepori pox v.
- louping ill v.
- Lunyo v.
- lymphocytic choriomeningitis v.
- lymphogranuloma venereum v.
- Marituba v.
- masked v.
- Mayaro v.
- measles v.
- Mengo v.
- MM v.
- molluscum contagiosum v.
- molluscum sebaceum v.
- monkey B v.
- mumps v.

virus *(continued)*
- Murray Valley encephalitis v.
- Newcastle disease v.
- nonbacterial gastroenteritis v.
- Norwalk v.
- Ntaya v.
- Omsk hemorrhagic fever v.
- O'nyong-nyong fever v.
- orf v.
- Oriboca v.
- ornithosis v.
- Oropouche v.
- orphan v.
- pappataci fever v.
- parainfluenza v., types 1, 2, 3, 4
- parapox v.
- parrot v.
- pharyngoconjunctival fever v.
- phlebotomus fever v.
- pneumonitis v.
- poliomyelitis v.
- polyoma v.
- Powassan v.
- pox v.
- psittacosis v.
- rabies v.
- respiratory exanthematous v.
- respiratory infection v.
- respiratory syncytial v.
- Rift Valley fever v.
- roseola infantum v.
- Rous sarcoma v.

Additional Entries

_____
_____
_____
_____

virus *(continued)*
    RS v.
    rubella v.
    rubeola v.
    Russian spring-summer
        encephalitis v.
    St. Louis encephalitis v.
    Salisbury common cold v.
    salivary gland v.
    sand-fly fever v.
    Semliki Forest v.
    Sendai v.
    serum hepatitis v.
    Simbu v.
    simian sarcoma v.
    Sindbis v.
    smallpox v.
    street v.
    Teschen v.
    Theiler's v.
    tickborne v.
    trachoma v.
    Uganda S v.
    unorganized v.
    Uruma v.
    vaccinia v.
    varicella v.
    varicella-zoster v.
    variola v.
    VEE v.
    verruca v.
    vesicular stomatitis v.
    WEE v.
    Wesselsbron v.
    West Nile v.
    Willowbrook v.
    yellow fever v.
    Zika v.

virus *(continued)*
    2060 v.
visceromegaly
viscidosis
vitreocapsulitis
vivax malaria
Vogt's syndrome
Vogt-Koyanagi disease
Vohwinkel's syndrome
Volkmann's
    contracture
    paralysis
Voltolini's disease
vomit
    Barcoo v.
    bilious v.
    black v.
    coffee-ground v.
vomiting
    cerebral v.
    cyclic v.
    dry v.
    fecal v.
    hysterical v.
    nervous v.
    periodic v.
    pernicious v.
    v. of pregnancy
    projectile v.
    recurrent v.
    stercoraceous v.
vomitus
von Bechterew's disease
von Gierke's disease
von Hippel-Lindau disease
von Hippel's disease
von Recklinghausen's disease
von Willebrand's disease

Additional Entries

VPC (ventricular premature contraction)
VPD (ventricular premature depolarization)
VRI (viral respiratory infection)
VSD (ventricular septal defect)
VSV (vesicular stomatitis virus)
VT (ventricular tachycardia)
vulvitis
    diabetic v.
    eczematiform v.
    erosive v.
    leukoplakic v.
    phlegmonous v.
    plasma cell v.
    pseudoleukoplakic v.
vulvovaginitis
    infectious pustular v.
    senile v.
VW (von Willebrand's disease)
VZV (varicella-zoster virus)

Additional Entries

W

Waardenburg's syndrome
Wagner's disease
Waldenstrom's
   macroglobulinemia
Wallenberg's syndrome
Wardrop's disease
Wartenberg's disease
Warthin's tumor
warty dyskeratosis
wasserhelle
   w. hyperplasia
Wassilieff's disease
Waterhouse-Friderichsen
   syndrome
Watsonius watsoni
WC (whooping cough)
WDLL (well-differentiated
   lymphocytic lymphoma)
WE (western encephalitis;
   western encephalomyelitis)
Weber-Christian disease
Wegener's granulomatosis
Wegner's disease
Weil-Marchesani syndrome
Weil's disease
Weir Mitchell's disease
Welch's bacillus
well-differentiated lymphocytic
   lymphoma
Wenckebach block
Werdnig-Hoffmann
   disease
   paralysis
Werlhof's disease
Wermer's syndrome

Werner's syndrome
Werner-His disease
Wernicke-Korsakoff syndrome
Wernicke-Mann hemiplegia
Wernicke's
   disease
   encephalopathy
   syndrome
Wesselsbron
   disease
   virus
Westermark's sign
West Nile fever
West Nile virus
Westphal's disease
Westphal-Strumpell
   pseudosclerosis
West's syndrome
Weyer's oligodactyly syndrome
Weyers-Thier syndrome
wheeze
whiplash
Whipple's disease
White's disease
Whitmore's
   bacillus
   disease
whooping cough
Whytt's disease
Wichmann's asthma
Widal's syndrome Widal-
   Abrami disease
Wilder's sign
Wildervanck syndrome
Wilkie's disease

Additional Entries

___
___
___
___
___

Willebrand's syndrome
Williams-Campbell syndrome
Williams syndrome
Willis' disease
Willowbrook virus
Wilms' tumor
Wilson-Mikity syndrome
Wilson's disease
Winckel's disease
Windscheid's disease
Winiwarter-Buerger disease
Winkler's disease
Winter's syndrome
Winton disease
wire-loop lesion
Wiskott-Aldrich syndrome
Witkop's disease
Witkop-Von Sallmann disease
WK (Wernicke-Korsakoff syndrome)
Wohlfahrtia
    W. magnifica
    W. opaca
    W. vigil
Wohlfart-Kugelberg-Welander disease
Wolff-Chaikoff effect
wolffian
    w. duct carcinoma
Wolff-Parkinson-White syndrome

Wolf-Hirschhorn syndrome
Wolfram syndrome
Wolman's disease
woolsorter's disease
Woringer-Kolopp disease
Wright's syndrome
wound
wound *(continued)*
    abraded w.
    avulsed w.
    contused w.
    gunshot w.
    incised w.
    lacerated w.
    missile w.
    mutilating w.
    penetrating w.
    perforating w.
    stab w.
    superficial w.
WPW (Wolff-Parkinson-White syndrome)
wrist
    tennis w.
Wuchereria
    W. bancrofti
    W. malayi
    W. pacifica
wuchereriasis

Additional Entries

X

xanthelasma
xanthinuria
xanthochromia
xanthogranuloma
    juvenile x.
xanthoma
    x. diabeticorum
    x. disseminatum
    eruptive x.
    juvenile x.
    x. striatum palmare
    x. tendinosum
    x. tuberosum simplex
xanthomatosis
    biliary hypercholesterolemic x.
    x. bulbi
    cerebrotendinous x.
    chronic idiopathic x. x. corneae
    x. generalisata ossium
    x. iridis
    primary familial x.
    Wolman x.
xanthomatous
Xanthomonas
xanthopsia
xanthopsis
xanthosarcoma
xanthurenic aciduria
xanthuria
XDP (xeroderma pigmentosum)
xenophthalmia
Xenopsylla
    X. astia
    X. brasiliensis
    X. cheopis
Xenopus
    X. laevis
xenorexia
xerocytosis
xeroderma
    x. pigmentosum
xerophthalmia
xerosis conjunctival x.
    corneal x.
    x. cutis
    x. parenchymatosa
    x. superficialis
xerostomia
xiphodynia
xiphoiditis
XP (xeroderma pigmentosum)
XT (exotropia)
XYZ syndrome

Additional Entries

Additional Entries

Y

yellow
    y. fever
    y. fever virus
Yersinia
    Y. enterocolitica

Yersinia *(continued)*
    Y. pestis
    Y. pseudotuberculosis
YF (yellow fever)
Yokogawa's fluke
Young's syndrome

Additional Entries

Additional Entries

Z

Zahn's infarct
Zahorsky's disease
Zaufal's sign
ZE (Zollinger-Ellison syndrome)
Zeeman's effect
Zellweger syndrome
Zenker's
    degeneration
    diverticulum
    dysplasia
Ziehen-Oppenheim disease
Zieve syndrome
Zika virus
Zollinger-Ellison syndrome
Zoogloea
Zoomastigophora
zoster
    z. sine eruptione
    ophthalmic z.
Zumbusch's psoriasis
zygomycosis
Zymobacterium
Zymomonas
zymosis

Additional Entries

Additional Entries

DISEASES

A accumulated.
Acosta's d.
Adam's d.
Adams-Stokes d.
d's of adaptation
Addison's d.
adult celiac d.
airsac d.
akamushi d.
Akureyri d.
Aland eye d.
Albers-Schonberg d.
Alexander's d.
alkali d.
allogeneic d.
Almeida's d.
Alper's d.
alpha chain d.
altitude d.
Alzheimer's d.
Anders' d.
Andersen's d.
Andes d.
anti-glomerular basement membrane antibody d.
Apert's d.
Apert-Crouzon d.
Aran-Duchenne d.
arc-welder's d.
Armstrong's d.
atopic d.
Australian X d.
autoimmune d.
aviators' d.
Ayerza's d.

Azorean d.

B Baastrup's d.
Baelz's d.
Bamberger's d.
Bamberger-Marie d.
Bang's d.
Bannister's d.
Barcoo d.
Barlow's d.
barometer-maker's d.
Barraquer's d.
Basedow's d.
Batten d.
bauxite workers' d.
Bayle's d.
Bazin's d.
Beard's d.
Beau's d.
Beauvais' d.
Beck's d.
Beguez Cesar d.
Behcet's d.
Behr's d.
Beigel's d.
Bekhterev's d.
Benson's d.
Berger's d.
Bergeron's d.
Berlin's d.
Bernard-Soulier d.
Bernhardt's d.
Bernhardt-Roth d.
Besnier-Boeck d.
Bettlach May d.

Additional Entries

Biedl's d.
Bielschowsky-Jansky d.
Biermer's d.
Bilderbeck's d.
Billroth's d.
Binswanger's d.
black d.
blinding filarial d.
Blocq's d.
Bloodgood's d.
Blount d. Boeck's d.
Borna d.
Bornholm d.
Bostock's d.
bottom d.
Bouchard's d.
Bouchet-Gsell d.
Bouillaud's d.
Bourneville's d.
Bouveret's d.
Bowen's d.
Bradley's d.
brancher glycogen storage d.
Breda's d.
Breisky's d.
Bright's d.
Brill's d.
Brill-Symmer d.
Brill-Zinsser d.
Brinton's d.
Brion-Kayser d.
broad-beta d.
Brodie's d.
bronzed d.
Brooke's d.
Brown-Sequard d.
Brown-Symmers d.
Bruck's d.

Brushfield-Wyatt d.
Bruton's d.
Budd-Chiari d.
Buerger's d.
Buerger-Grutz d.
buffalo d.
Buhl's d.
Buschke's d.
bush d.
Busquet's d.
Buss d.
Busse-Bushchke d.

C Cacchi-Ricci d.
Caffey's d.
California d.
caloric d.
Calve-Perthes d.
Camurati-Engelmann d.
Canavan's d.
Caroli's d.
Carrion's d.
Castellani's d.
cat-scratch d.
Calvare's d.
celiac d.
central core of muscle d.
Chaber's d.
Chagas' d.
Charcot's d.
Charcot-Marie-Tooth d.
Charlouis' d.
Chediak-Higashi d.
Chester's d.
Chiari's d.
Chiari-Frommel d.
Chicago d.

Additional Entries

cholesteryl ester storage d. (CESD)
Christian's d.
chronic granulomatous d.
chronic obstructive pulmonary d. (COPD)
circling d.
climatic d.
Coats' d.
Cogan's d.
cold agglutinin d.
collagen d.
combined immunodeficiency d.
combined system d.
communicable d.
complicating d.
compressed-air d.
Concato's d.
Conor and Bruch's d.
Conradi's d.
constitutional d.
contagious d.
Cooley's d.
Corbus' d.
Cori's d.
cornstalk d.
corridor d.
Corrigan's d.
Corvisart's d.
Cotugno's d.
covering d.
Cowden's d.
Creutzfeldt-Jakob d.
Crigler-Najjar d.
Crocq's d.
Crohn's d.
Crouzon's d.
Cruveilhier's

Cruz-Chagas d.
Csillag's d.
Cushing's d.
cystic d. of breast
cystic d. of lung
cysticercus d.
cystine d.
cytomegalic inclusion d.
Czerny's d.

D Daae's d.
Dalrymple's d.
Danlos' d.
Darling's d.
David's d.
debrancher glycogen storage d.
degenerative joint d.
Degos' d.
Dejerine's d.
demyelinating d.
dense deposit d.
deprivation d.
de Quervain's d.
Dercum's d.
dermopathic herpesvirus d.
Deutschlander's d.
Devic's d.
diamond-skin d.
diverticular d.
Dohle d.
Down's d.
Dubin-Sprinz d.
Dubini's d.
Dubois' d.
Duchenne's d.
Duchenne-Aran d.
Duchenne-Griesinger d.
Duhring's d.

Additional Entries

DISEASES, FURSTNER'S D. / **291**

Dukes' d.
Duncan's d.
Dupre's d.
Durand-Nicolas-Favre d.
Durante's d.

E Eales d.
Ebola virus d.
Ebstein's d.
echinococcus d.
Economo's d.
Eddowes' d.
Edsall's d.
Ehlers-Danlos d.
endemic d.
Engelmann's d.
Engel-Recklinghausen d.
English d.
English sweating d.
eosinophilic endomyocardial d.
epidemic d.
Epstein's d.
Erb's d.
Erb-Charcot d.
Erb-Goldflam d.
Erb-Landouzy d.
Eulenburg's d.
extensor process d.
extrapyramidal d.

F Fabry's d.
Fahr-Volhard d.
Fallot's d.
Fanconi's d.
Farber d.
fat-deficiency d.
Fauchard d.

Favre-Durand-Nicholas d.
Feer's d.
Fenwick's d.
fibrocystic d.
fibrocystic d. of the pancreas
Fiedler's d.
fifth venereal d.
Filatov's d.
Filatov-Dukes d.
file-cutters' d. fish-slime d.
Flajani's d.
Flatau-Schilder d.
flax-dresser's d.
Flegel's d.
Fleischner's d.
flint d.
fluke d.
focal d.
foot-and-mouth d.
Forbes' d.
Fordyce's d.
Forestier d.
Forster's d.
Fothergill's d.
Fournier's d.
fourth venereal d.
Fox-Fordyce d.
Francis' d.
Frankl-Hochwart's d.
Frei's d.
Freiberg's d.
Friedlander's d.
Friedreich's d.
Frommel's d.
functional d.
functional cardiovascular d.
Furstner's d.

Additional Entries

DISEASES, Gaisbock's d. / **292**

GGaisbock's d.
gamma chain d.
Gamna's d.
Gamstorp's d.
Gandy-Nanta d.
gannister d.
Garre's d.
Gaucher's d.
Gee's d.
Gee-Thaysen d.
genetic d.
Gerhardt's d.
Gerlier's d.
giant platelet d.
Gibney's d.
Gierke's d.
Gilbert's d.
Gilchrist's d.
Gilles de la Tourette's d.
Glanzmann's d.
Glasser's d.
Glenard's d.
Glisson's d.
glucose-6-phosphatase
   dehydrogenase d.
glycogen storage d.
Goldflam's d.
Goldstein's d.
Gorham's d.
Graefe's d.
graft-versus-host d.
Grave's d.
Greenfield's d.
Gross' d.
Grover's d.
Guinon's d.
Gull's d.
Gumboro d.

Gunther's d.

HHabermann's d.
Haff d.
Haglund's d.
Hagner's d.
Hailey-Hailey d.
Hallervorden-Spatz d.
Hallopeau's d.
Hall's d.
Hamman's d.
Hammond's d.
Hand's d.
hand-foot-and-mouth d.
Hand-Schuller-Christian d.
Hanot's d.
Hansen's d.
d. of the Hapsburgs
Harada's d.
Hartnup d.
Hashimoto's d.
heart d.
heartwater d.
heavy-chain d.
Heberden's d.
Hebra's d.
Heerfordt's d.
Heine-Medin d.
Heller-Dohle d.
helminthic d.
hemoglobin d.
hemoglobin C-thalassemia d.
hemoglobin E-thalassemia d.
hemolytic d. of newborn
hemorrhagic d. of the newborn
Henderson-Jones d.
hepatolenticular d.
hepatorenal glycogen storage d.

Additional Entries

_____
_____
_____
_____

hereditary d.
heredoconstitutional d.
heredodegenerative d.
Herlitz's d.
Hers' d.
Herter's d.
Heubner's d.
hip-joint d.
Hippel's d.
Hippel-Lindau d.
Hirschsprung's d.
His d.
hock d.
Hodgkin's d.
Hodgson's d.
Hoffa's d.
holoendemic d.
hoof-and-mouth d.
hookworm d.
Horton's d.
Huchard's d.
Hunt's d.
Huntington d.
Hurler's d.
Hutchinson's d.
Hutchinson-Gilford d.
Hutinel's d.
hyaline membrane d.
hydatid d.
hydatid d., alveolar
hydatid d., unilocular
hydrocephaloid d.
hyperendemic d.
hypopigmentation-
   immunodeficiency d.

I I-cell d.
idiopathic d.

immune-complex d's
immunodeficiency d.
immunoproliferative small
   intestine d.
inclusion d.
infantile celiac d.
infectious d.
inflammatory bowel d.
inherited d.
interstitial lung d.
Isambert's d.
Isle of Wight d.
itch d.

J Jaffe-Lichtenstein d.
Jakob-Creutzfeldt d.
Jaksch's d.
Janet's d.
Jansen's d.
Johne's d.
Johnson-Stevens d.
Joseph d.
jumping d.
juvenile Paget d.

K Kahler's d.
Kaiserstuhl d.
Kaschin-Beck d.
Kashin-Beck d.
Katayama d.
Kawasaki d.
Keshan d.
Kienbock's d.
Kimura's d.
Kinnier Wilson d.
Kirkland's d.
kissing d.
Klebs' d.

Additional Entries

_____
_____
_____
_____
_____

Klemperer's d.
Klippel's d.
knight's d.
Kohler's bone d.
Kohler's second d.
Kohler-Pellegrini-Stieda d.
Krishaber's d.
Kufs' d.
Kugelberg-Welander d.
Kuhnt-Junius d.
Kummell's d.
Kummell-Verneuil d.
Kyasanur Forest d.
Kyrle's d.

L Laennec's d.
Lafora's d.
Lancereaux-Mathieu d.
Landouzy's d.
Landry's d.
Lane's d.
Larsen's d.
Lauber's d.
Leber's d.
Legal's d.
Legg-Calve d.
legionnaires' d.
Leigh d.
Leiner's d.
Lenegre's d.
Leriche's d.
Letterer-Siwe d.
Lev's d.
Lewandowsky-Lutz d.
Leyden's d.
Libman-Sacks d.
Lichtheim's d.
Lignac-Fanconi d.

Lindau's d.
lipid storage d.
Lobo's d.
Lobstein's d.
local d.
Lorain's d.
Lowe's d.
Luft's d.
lumpy skin d.
lung fluke d.
lunger d.
Lutembacher's d.
Lutz-Splendore-Almeida d.
Lyell's d.
Lyme d.
lysosomal storage d.

M McArdle's d.
Machado-Joseph d.
Mackenzie's d.
MacLean-Maxwell d.
Madelung's d.
Maher's d.
Majocchi's d.
Malassez's d.
Malibu d.
Manson's d.
maple bark d.
maple syrup urine d.
Marburg d.
March's d.
Marchiafava-Bignami d.
Marchiafava-Micheli d.
Marek's d.
Marie's d.
Marie-Bamberger d.
Marie-Strumpell d.
Marie-Tooth d.

Additional Entries

Marion's d.
Marsh's d.
Martin's d.
Medin's d.
Mediterranean d.
medullary cystic d.
Meige's d.
Meleda d.
Menetrier's d.
Meniere's d.
Menkes' d.
mental d.
Merzbacher-Pelizaeus d.
metabolic d.
metazoan d.
Meyer's d.
Meyer-Betz d.
microdrepanocytic d.
Mikulicz's d.
milky d.
Miller's d.
Mills' d.
Milroy's d.
Milton's d.
Minamata d.
Minor's d.
Mitchell's d.
mixed connective tissue d.
Mobius d.
Moeller-Barlow d.
molecular d.
Molten's d.
Mondor's d.
Monge's d.
Morel-Kraepelin d.
Morgagni's d.
Morquio-Brailsford d.
Morquio's d.

Morqui-Ullrich d.
Morton's d.
Morvan's d.
Moschcowitz's d.
motor neuron d.
mountain d.
moyamoya d.
Mozer's d.
mu chain d.
Mucha's d.
mucosal d.
mule spinner's d.
Munchmeyer's d.
Murray Valley d.
mushroom worker's d.

N Nairobi d.
nanukayami d.
navicular d.
Newcastle d.
Nicolas-Favre d.
Niemann d.
Norrie's d.
Norum-Gjone d.

O oasthouse urine d.
occupational d.
Oguchi's d.
Ohara's d. oid-oid d.
Ollier's d.
Ondiri d.
Opitz's d.
Oppenheim's d.
organic d.
Oriental lung fluke d.
Ormond's d.
Osgood-Schlatter d.
Osler's d.

Additional Entries

Osler-Vaquez d.
Osler-Weber-Rendu d.
Otto's d.
overeating d.
Owren's d.

P Paas's d.
Paget d.
Paget's d., extramammary
Panner's d.
parenchymatous d.
Parkinson's d.
Parrot's d.
Parry's d.
Patella's d.
Pavy's d.
Payr's d.
pearl-worker's d.
Pel-Ebstein d.
Pelizaeus-Merzbacher d.
Pellegrini's d.
pelvic inflammatory d.
peridontal d.
Perrin-Ferraton d.
Perthes' d.
Peyronie's d.
Pfeiffer's d.
Phocas' d.
phytanic acid storage d.
Pick's d.
Pictou d.
pink d.
Pinkus' d.
plaster-of-Paris d.
Plummer's d.
pneumatic hammer d.
policeman's d.
polycystic d. of kidneys

polycystic ovary d.
polycystic renal d.
polyendocrine autoimmune d.
Pompe's d.
Poncet's d.
Portuguese-Azorean d.
Posada-Wernicke d.
Pott's d.
pregnancy d.
Preiser's d.
Pringle's d.
Profichet's d.
pulseless d.
Purtscher's d.
Pyle's d.
pyramidal d.

Q Quervain's d.
Quincke's d.

R ragpicker's d.
Ramsay Hunt d.
rat-bite d.
Raynaud's d.
Recklinghausen's d.
Recklinghausen-Applebaum d.
Reclus' d.
redwater d.
Reed-Hodgkin d.
Refsum d.
Reiter's d.
Rendu-Osler-Weber d.
reportable d.
rheumatic heart d.
rheumatoid d.
Ribas-Torres d.
rice d.
Riedel's d.

Additional Entries

Riga-Fede d.
Riggs' d.
Ritter's d.
Robles' d.
Roger's d.
rolling d.
Romberg's d.
rose d.
Rossbach's d.
Rot's d.
Roth's d.
Roth-Bernhardt d.
Rougnon-Heberden d.
Roussy-Levy's d.
Rubarth's d.
Rummo's d.
Rust's d.
Ruysch's d.

S saccharine d.
Sach's d.
sacroiliac d.
St. Agatha's d.
St. Aignon's d.
St. Anthony's d.
St. Appolonia's d.
St. Avertin's d.
St. Blasius' d.
St. Dymphna's d.
St. Erasmus' d.
St. Fiacre's d.
St. Gervasius' d.
St. Gotthard's tunnel d.
St. Hubert's d.
St. Job's d.
St. Mathurin's d.
St. Modestus' d.
St. Roch's d.

St. Sement's d.
St. Valentine's d.
St. Zachary's d.
salivary gland d.
Sanders' d.
Sandhoff's d.
sandworm d.
San Joaquin Valley d.
Saunder's d.
Schamberg's d. Schanz's d.
Schaumann's d.
Scheuermann's d.
Schilder's d.
Schimmelbusch's d.
Schlatter's d.
Schmorl's d.
Scholz's d.
Schonlein's d.
Schonlein-Henoch d.
Schottmuller's d.
Schroeder's d.
Schuller's d.
Schuller-Christian d.
Schultz's d.
Schwediauer's d.
secondary d.
Seitelberger's d.
self-limited d.
Selter's d.
senecio d.
septic d.
serum d.
Sever's d.
severe combined
   immunodeficiency d.
sexually transmitted d.
Shaver's d.
shimamushi d.

Additional Entries
.

shuttlemaker's d.
sickle-cell d.
sickle cell-hemoglobin C d.
sickle cell-hemoglobin D d.
sickle cell-thalassemia d.
silo-filler's d.
Simmonds' d.
Simons' d.
sixth d.
sixth venereal d.
Sjogren's d.
Skevas-Zerfus d.
sleeping d.
Sly d.
Smith-Strang d.
Sneddon-Wilkinson d.
sod d.
specific d.
Spencer's d.
Spielmeyer-Vogt d.
sponge-diver's d.
Stargardt's d.
Steinert's d.
sterility d. Sternberg's d.
Sticker's d.
Stieda's d.
Still's d.
Stokes-Adams d.
Stokvis'd .
storage d.
storage pool d.
structural d.
Strumpell's d.
Strumpell-Leichtenstern d.
Strumpell-Lorain d.
Strumpell-Marie d.
Sturge's d.
Stuttgart d.

Sudeck's d.
Sutton's d.
Swift's d.
Swift-Feer d.
swineherd's d.
Sydenham's d.
Sylvest's d.
Symmers' d.
systemic d.

TTakahara's d.
Takayasu's d.
Talfan d.
Talma's d.
Tangier d.
tartaric d.
Tarui d.
Tay's d.
Tay-Sachs d.
Teschen d.
thalassemia-sickle cell d.
Thaysen's d.
Theiler's d.
Thiemann's d.
Thomsen's d.
Thomson's d.
thyrocardiac d.
thyrotoxic heart d.
Tietze's d.
Tillaux's d.
Tommaselli's d.
Tooth d.
Tornwaldt's d.
Tourette's d.
Trevor's d.
trophoblastic d.
tsutsugamushi d.
twist d.

Additional Entries

_____
_____
_____
_____

Tyzzer's d.
Tzaneen d.

U Underwood's d.
Unna-Thost d.
Unverricht's d.
Urbach-Wiethe d.

V vagabond's d.
van Bogaert's d.
van Buren's d.
Vaquez's d.
veldt d.
venereal d.
veno-occlusive d. of liver
Verneuil's d.
Verse's d.
vibration d.
Vidal's d.
Vincent's d.
Virchow's d.
Vogt's d.
Vogt-Spielmeyer d.
Volkmann's d.
Voltolini's d.
von Bechterew's d.
von Economo's d.
von Gierke's d.
von Hippel's d.
von Hippel-Lindau d.
von Jaksch's d.
von Meyenburg's d.
von Recklinghausen's d.
von Willebrand's d.
Vrolik's d.

W Wagner's d.
Waldenstrom's d.

Wallenberg's d.
Wardrop's d.
Wartenberg's d.
Wassilieff's d.
wasting d.
Weber-Christian d.
Weber-Dimitri d.
Weber's d.
Weber-Christian d.
Wegner's d.
Weil's d.
Weir Mitchell's d.
Werdnig-Hoffmann d.
Werlhof's d.
Werner-His d.
Werner-Schultz d.
Wernicke's d.
Wesselsbron d.
Westphal-Strumpell d.
Whipple's d.
White's d.
Whitmore's d.
Whytt's d.
Wilkie's d.
Willis' d.
Wilson's d.
Winckel's d.
Windscheid's d.
Winiwarter-Buerger d.
Winkler's d.
Winton d.
Witkop's d.
Wohlfart-Kugelberg-Welander d.
Wolman's d.
woolsorters' d.
Woringer-Kolopp d.

Additional Entries

DISEASES, X D. / **300**

X x d.
X-linked lymphoproliferative d.

Z Zahorsky's d.
Ziehen-Oppenheim d.

Additional Entries

Ref
RB
115
S53

Shaw, Diane L.
Pathophysiologic word book.

$17.95

DATE

REFERENCE

DO NOT REMOVE FROM LIBRARY

SOUTH COLLEGE
709 Mall Blvd.
Savannah, GA 31406

BAKER & TAYLOR BOOKS